THE
EVERYTHING®
LOW-CARB
COOKBOOK

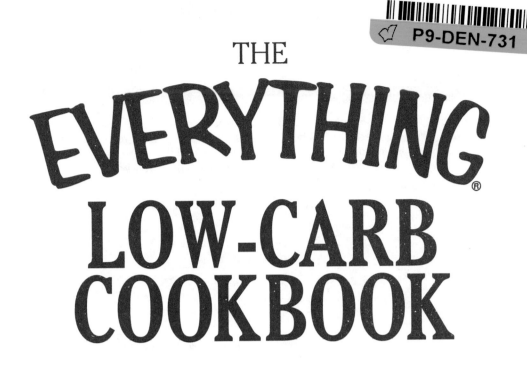

300 delicious recipes
to help reduce your carbohydrates
and stay healthy

Patricia M. Butkus

Adams Media Corporation
Avon, Massachusetts

EDITORIAL
Publishing Director: Gary M. Krebs
Managing Editor: Kate McBride
Copy Chief: Laura MacLaughlin
Acquisitions Editor: Bethany Brown
Development Editor: Karen Johnson Jacot
Production Editor: Khrysti Nazzaro

PRODUCTION
Production Director: Susan Beale
Production Manager: Michelle Roy Kelly
Series Designers: Daria Perreault and Colleen Cunningham
Layout and Graphics: Colleen Cunningham,
Rachael Eiben, Michelle Roy Kelly,
Daria Perreault, Erin Ring

An Everything® Series Book.
Everything® is a registered trademark of Adams Media Corporation.

Published by Adams Media Corporation
57 Littlefield Street, Avon, MA 02322 U.S.A.
www.adamsmedia.com

ISBN: 1-58062-784-6
Printed in the United States of America.

J I H G F E D C

Library of Congress Cataloging-in-Publication Data
Butkus, Patricia M.
The everything low-carb cookbook / Patricia M. Butkus.
p.   cm.   -- (An everything series book)
ISBN 1-58062-784-6
1. Low-carbohydrate diet–Recipes. I. Title. II. Everything series.
RM237.73   .B88 2003
641.5'638–dc21

2002014284

The Everything® Low-Carb Cookbook is intended as a reference volume only, not as a medical manual. In light of the complex, individual, and specific nature of health problems, this book is not intended to replace professional medical advice. The ideas, procedures, and suggestions in this book are intended to supplement, not replace, the advice of a trained medical professional. Consult your physician before adopting the suggestions in this books, as well as about any condition that may require diagnosis or medical attention. The authors and publisher disclaim any liability arising directly or indirectly from the use of this book.

This publication is designed to provide accurate and authoritative information with regard to the subject matter covered. It is sold with the understanding that the publisher is not engaged in rendering legal, accounting, or other professional advice. If legal advice or other expert assistance is required, the services of a competent professional person should be sought.
—From a *Declaration of Principles* jointly adopted by a Committee of the American Bar Association and a Committee of Publishers and Associations

Illustrations by Barry Littmann.

This book is available at quantity discounts for bulk purchases.
For information, call 1-800-872-5627.

Visit the entire Everything® series at everything.com

Contents

INTRODUCTION V

CHAPTER 1 *Easy Appetizers* 1

CHAPTER 2 *Five or Fewer Ingredients* 17

CHAPTER 3 *French Entrées* 33

CHAPTER 4 *Italian Food* 53

CHAPTER 5 *Mexican Specialties* 69

CHAPTER 6 *Fusion Fun* 79

CHAPTER 7 *Salads and Dressings* 95

CHAPTER 8 *Soups and Stews* 113

CHAPTER 9 *Sides* 129

CHAPTER 10 *Lunch* 151

CHAPTER 11 *Comfort Food* 177

CHAPTER 12 *Breakfast* 191

CHAPTER 13 *Desserts* 203

CHAPTER 14 *Weekend Meals* 217

CHAPTER 15 *Entertaining* 255

CHAPTER 16 *Holiday Dishes* 279

APPENDIX A *Easy Dishes at a Glance* 302

INDEX 305

Introduction

WELCOME TO THE WORLD OF LOW-CARB COOKING! There are many reasons why you might choose to decrease the number of carbohydrates you consume. Whether it's a choice based on dietary needs or a weight-loss plan, *The Everything® Low-Carb Cookbook* is the perfect cookbook to help you reduce your carbohydrate intake. Different people have different dietary needs, and they are as varied as the recipes in this book. This book offers you more than 300 great-tasting recipes that are low in carbohydrates but not low on flavor.

What Is a Carbohydrate?

In a word, fuel. All energy in food comes from carbohydrates, proteins, or fatty acids. Carbohydrates are high-energy chemical compounds that are found in foods like breads, pasta, cereal, and vegetables. There are two types of carbohydrates—sugars (also called simple carbohydrates) and starches (or complex carbohydrates).

Simple sugars are absorbed directly into the bloodstream fairly quickly after you eat them. That's why you get a quick burst of energy from a candy bar, followed by a crash as your blood sugar level drops once the sugars are absorbed.

Starches are digested into simpler sugars, which are further converted into glucose. Glucose is the main source of energy for the cells of the human body. Because it takes longer for the body to break down and digest these carbohydrates, the sugars enter the bloodstream at a fairly constant rate.

Your body uses the energy it needs and stores the rest for later use. When you eat more carbs than your body needs, the high glucose levels cause your body to produce more fat to store the excess energy.

Diets that consistently contain more carbohydrates than the body needs can lead to health problems such as obesity and, in some cases, diabetes. Research has also suggested that diets high in starch contribute to atherosclerosis and heart disease, the number one cause of death in the United States.

So while it is important to have carbohydrates in your diet, controlling your intake to reasonable levels is always smart. *The Everything® Low-Carb Cookbook* gives you over 300 recipes for every occasion that will keep you low on carbs but high on taste!

Nutritional Analyses

Every recipe is rated to reflect the carbohydrate amount and includes specific carb counts. Using a reputable, nationally recognized computerized nutritional analysis program, I determined the total carb count on a per serving basis. Several of the current popular programs for calculating carbs subtract the fiber content before reporting the carb count. My analysis is based on the full carb amount; no compensations have been made. If you're counting net carbs, recipes containing ingredients with fiber will have lower carb counts than indicated here.

It's very difficult to determine accurate fat content in final recipes, especially given that much of the fat used during cooking doesn't remain in the final dish. Keep in mind that 1 gram of fat equals 9 calories.

You will notice two ratings used throughout the book for each recipe. Every recipe has a carb level identified as "Low" or "Moderate." Although the moderate recipes have a higher level of carbohydrates, they are still low-carb recipes.

- **LOW**—These recipes all contain 10 grams or fewer of carbohydrates per serving
- **MODERATE**—These recipes all contain between 10 and 20 grams of carbohydrates per serving

Eating healthy is an important part of your lifestyle. These recipes make it easy to eat well while still controlling your carb intake. Enjoy.

CHAPTER 1

Easy Appetizers

Party Cheese Balls ❖   2

Jicama and Chorizo Chips ❖   2

Crabmeat on Red Pepper Strips ❖   3

Hot Artichoke Dip ❖   3

Spinach and Ricotta Dip ❖   4

Mushrooms with Mediterranean Stuffing ❖   4

Spicy Jicama Chips ❖   5

Ham Cornets ❖   5

Portobello Mushrooms with Warm Garlic Flan   6

Artichoke Bottoms with Herbed Cheese ❖   7

Parmesan Crisps ❖   7

Caponata ❖   8

Grilled Pineapple and Avocado Chutney ❖   9

Olive Tapanade ❖   10

Mock Caviar ❖   10

Pesto Eggplant Caviar   11

Asian-Style Paste ❖   12

Jalapeño Paste ❖   12

Sausage Appetizers ❖   13

Basic Party Dip and Five Variations ❖   14

Warm Spinach and Artichoke Dip ❖   16

❖ **Indicates Easy Recipe** ❖

Party Cheese Balls

Serves 25
Carb Level: Low

Per serving:

Carbohydrate:	2.1 g
Protein:	8.0 g

This recipe produces 2 balls—keep 1 in the freezer for surprise get-togethers.

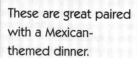

8 ounces cream cheese, softened
12 ounces blue cheese, crumbled
1 pound sharp Cheddar cheese, shredded
1 tablespoon Worcestershire sauce
2 tablespoons finely minced onion
Salt and white pepper to taste
1 cup pecan chips, toasted

Using a wooden spoon or food processor, mix together all the ingredients, *except* the pecan chips, until smooth. Shape the mixture into 2 balls, about 1 pound each. Roll each ball in the pecan chips to coat. Chill quickly. Keep in the refrigerator and serve chilled. The extra ball may be stored in the freezer, double wrapped in plastic film, for up to 1 month.

Jicama and Chorizo Chips

Serves 10
Carb Level: Low

Per serving:

Carbohydrate:	6.1 g
Protein:	9.3 g

These are great paired with a Mexican-themed dinner.

6 ounces goat cheese, softened
5 ounces spicy salsa
½ pound chorizo sausage
1 medium jicama, peeled, quartered, and sliced
Salt and white pepper to taste
Cilantro leaves for garnish

1. Combine the goat cheese and salsa in a small bowl. Use the tines of a fork to blend until incorporated; set aside. Slice the chorizo into ⅛-inch-thick slices. Heat a nonstick sauté pan over medium-high heat. Add the chorizo and cook, uncovered, until lightly browned on both sides. Remove with a slotted spoon to paper towels.
2. To assemble, place about ¾ teaspoon goat cheese mixture on each jicama chip. Top with a slice of the browned chorizo and garnish with fresh cilantro leaves. Serve immediately.

Crabmeat on Red Pepper Strips

Serves 4

Carb Level: Low

Per serving:

Carbohydrate:	9.6 g
Protein:	11.8 g

Serve in individual strips as an appetizer or place 3 strips on a bed of greens as a starter course.

∿

⅓ cup mayonnaise
2 green onions, finely chopped
½ plum tomato, seeded and
*   minced*
2 tablespoons chopped fresh
*   parsley and tarragon combined*
2 teaspoon fresh lemon juice
½ teaspoon grated fresh lemon zest

Pinch of cayenne pepper
8 ounces crabmeat, flaked (about
*   2 cups lightly packed)*
Salt and freshly ground black
*   pepper to taste*
2 large yellow, red, or green bell
*   peppers, cut into 1" × 2" strips*
Fresh chervil sprigs for garnish

Mix together the mayonnaise, green onions, tomato, chopped parsley and tarragon, lemon juice, lemon zest, and cayenne in a medium-size bowl until blended. Add the crabmeat and toss lightly to coat. Season with salt and pepper. Spoon 1 or 2 teaspoons of crab mixture onto each bell pepper strip. Garnish with chervil sprigs.

Hot Artichoke Dip

Serves 10

Carb Level: Low

Per serving:

Carbohydrate:	5.0 g
Protein:	2.1 g

Try this recipe with the guilt-free Jicama Chips for a perfect pairing.

∿

1 (10 ¾-ounce) can artichoke
*   hearts, rinsed, drained, and*
*   chopped*
2 cloves garlic, minced
¼ cup mayonnaise

Dash of Worcestershire sauce
½ cup grated Parmesan cheese
Salt and white pepper to taste

1. Preheat oven to 350°.
2. Combine all the ingredients in a 2-quart ovenproof glass dish and bake, uncovered, for 25 minutes. Serve hot with crisps or vegetable chips.

Spinach and Ricotta Dip

Serves 12

Carb Level: Low

Per serving:

Carbohydrate:	2.1 g
Protein:	0.9 g

This is a great party recipe—easy to make ahead and easy to transport.

1 (10-ounce) package frozen
   chopped spinach, thawed
   and drained
½ cup ricotta cheese
⅓ cup mayonnaise
¼ cup chopped green onions
¼ cup sour cream
3 tablespoons lemon juice

2 tablespoons grated onion
   (including juice)
Dash of Worcestershire sauce
Salt and freshly ground black
   pepper to taste
Chopped parsley for garnish

Combine all the ingredients, *except* the parsley, in a food processor and pulse until smooth. Adjust seasoning to taste. Transfer to a bowl and chill thoroughly. Top with chopped parsley. Serve with fresh trimmed vegetables or toasted bread rounds.

Mushrooms with Mediterranean Stuffing

Serves 10
(about 30 mushrooms)

Carb Level: Low

Per serving:

Carbohydrate:	3.0 g
Protein:	2.7 g

Everyone loves no-cook recipes during the summer. This is a favorite for an easy do-ahead preparation.

⅔ cup low-fat cottage cheese
3 ounces feta cheese, crumbled
2 tablespoons freshly snipped
   dill
1 teaspoon lemon juice
½ teaspoon olive oil

½ teaspoon dried oregano
Salt to taste
30 medium mushroom caps,
   cleaned and stemmed
Fresh dill sprigs for garnish

Combine the first 7 ingredients in a small bowl and mix until blended thoroughly. Spoon about 1 teaspoon of filling into each mushroom cap. Garnish with fresh dill sprigs and serve.

Spicy Jicama Chips

*1 jicama, peeled, quartered,
  and thinly sliced*
*⅓ cup freshly squeezed
  lime juice*

1 teaspoon chili powder
½ teaspoon ground red pepper
Salt to taste

Place the jicama slices in shallow glass dish and toss with lime juice; allow to marinate for 30 minutes at room temperature. Drain the chips and transfer to a serving platter; sprinkle with chili powder, pepper, and salt. Serve immediately with your favorite dip.

Serves 10	
Carb Level: Low	
Per serving:	
Carbohydrate:	2.2 g
Protein:	0.3 g

Cool crispy jicama chips are a great alternative to potato chips. Use these chips as a base for canapés— also great with Mexican dips.

Ham Cornets

*8 ounces cream cheese,
  softened*
1 tablespoon Dijon mustard
*2 tablespoons chopped fresh
  tarragon*

*Salt and freshly ground black
  pepper to taste*
*10 slices good-quality deli ham,
  cut into thirds*
30 water crackers

Mix together the cream cheese, Dijon, tarragon, and salt and pepper in a small bowl until blended. Place about ¾ teaspoon of the cream cheese mixture at the short end of a ham slice and roll into a cornet shape. Repeat with the remaining slices, reserving a small amount of the cream cheese mixture. To assemble, smear a very small amount of the cream cheese mixture on each cracker as a "glue" to secure the ham cornet. Top each cracker with the cornet and serve immediately.

Serves 15	
Carb Level: Low	
Per serving:	
Carbohydrate:	7.6 g
Protein:	17.8 g

A quick stop at the deli counter and you're ready with the main ingredient for these savory bites.

Portobello Mushrooms with Warm Garlic Flan

Serves 6

Carb Level: Low

Per serving:

Carbohydrate:	6.4 g
Protein:	14.0 g

This is a dressy first course worthy of an intimate dinner with good friends.

∾

6 portobello mushrooms
4 teaspoons chopped chives
   or garnish

Marinade:
1 cup olive oil
2 cloves garlic, minced
1 tablespoon finely chopped
   fresh rosemary
1 tablespoon finely chopped
   fresh oregano
1 tablespoon finely chopped
   fresh basil
Juice of 1 lemon
2 teaspoons salt

1 teaspoon black pepper
3 tablespoons balsamic vinegar
2 teaspoons soy sauce

Garlic flan:
1 cup heavy cream
3 cloves roasted garlic,
   cut in half
3 egg yolks
1 teaspoon powdered,
   unflavored gelatin
Pinch of salt
Pinch of white pepper
Grating of fresh nutmeg
Butter, softened

1. Remove and discard the stems from the mushrooms. Clean the caps using a damp paper towel.
2. In a medium-size bowl, whisk together all of the marinade ingredients. Add the mushroom caps and let sit, uncovered, for 2 hours at room temperature.
3. Preheat the broiler or the grill to high heat.
4. Broil or grill the mushrooms for about 3 minutes on each side; let cool. Cut the mushrooms into ½-inch slices and set aside.
5. Preheat the oven to 350°.
6. To prepare the flan: Bring the cream and garlic to a simmer in a small saucepan over medium-low heat. Transfer the mixture to a blender or food processor and add the egg yolks, gelatin, salt, pepper, and nutmeg; purée until smooth.
7. Using 4-ounce buttered ramekins, pour in the custard to the top. Place the ramekins in a baking pan and fill it with ½ inch of water. Bake for about 1 hour or until the custard is set.
8. Position each ramekin in the center of a salad plate. Serve the slices of mushroom around the flan and garnish with chopped chives.

Artichoke Bottoms with Herbed Cheese

1 can artichoke bottoms, rinsed and drained
8 ounces cream cheese, softened
2 tablespoons chopped fresh herbs (parsley, basil, chives, etc.)
Salt and freshly ground black pepper to taste
30 fresh radish slices

Slice the artichoke bottoms into 30 neatly trimmed slices. Mix together the cream cheese, herbs, and salt and pepper in a small bowl until smooth. Use a pastry bag to pipe a small rosette of the cream cheese mixture (about 1 rounded tablespoon each) onto each artichoke slice. Top with a radish slice and serve immediately.

Serves 15

Carb Level: Low

Per serving:

Carbohydrate:	1.0 g
Protein:	1.3 g

Canned artichoke bottoms are a great item to have on hand when you need a quick appetizer with an elegant look.

Parmesan Crisps

1 cup shredded (not grated) Parmesan cheese
Freshly ground black pepper to taste

1. Preheat oven to 325°. Line a cookie sheet with parchment paper.
2. Place rounded teaspoons of the shredded cheese on the parchment, equally spaced with about 2 to 2½ inches between each mound. Lightly flatten each mound with your fingertips to a circle about 1½ inches across. Sprinkle with pepper. Bake, checking after 3 minutes until the cheese just starts to melt and very lightly begins to brown. Remove immediately and transfer the crisps to a rack to cool. Store in airtight containers.

Serves 15

Carb Level: Low

Per serving:

Carbohydrate:	0.2 g
Protein:	2.2 g

Check the crisps frequently while baking—the color should just start to turn golden. Overcooked cheese has a bitter aftertaste.

Caponata

½ cup olive oil
6 medium zucchini, cut into
  ½-inch pieces
2 cups medium-diced onions
1 red pepper, seeded,
  medium dice
6 cloves garlic, peeled and
  finely chopped
2 cups diced fresh tomatoes
½ cup tomato purée
¼ cup capers, drained

¼ cup balsamic vinegar
Salt and freshly ground black
  pepper to taste
½ cup coarsely chopped
  walnuts, toasted

Heat the oil in a large nonstick sauté pan over medium-high heat. Add the zucchini and cook, stirring frequently, until lightly browned on all sides, about 5 minutes. Add all the remaining ingredients *except* the nuts and simmer for about 15 minutes, stirring frequently to prevent sticking. Season to taste, cool, and transfer to a glass or ceramic serving bowl. Cover and refrigerate overnight. Serve at room temperature, garnished with the walnuts.

Grilled Pineapple and Avocado Chutney

1 pineapple, peeled, cored, and cut into 1-inch-thick rings
1½ tablespoons vegetable oil
Salt and freshly ground black pepper to taste
2 small avocados, halved, pitted, and cut into ½-inch chunks
3 tablespoons fresh-squeezed lime juice
1 tablespoon jalapeño pepper, minced and seeded (about 1 small pepper)
¼ cup coarsely chopped fresh cilantro leaves

Serves 8
Carb Level: Moderate

Per serving:	
Carbohydrate:	11.6 g
Protein:	1.3 g

Serve the chutney the same day it is prepared (or the avocado will discolor).

∾

1. Prepare a charcoal grill or preheat a gas grill to high. Make sure the grill grate is clean and lightly oiled to prevent sticking. You can also use an indoor grill pan for this recipe.
2. Brush the pineapple rings lightly with oil and season with salt and pepper. Place on the grill for about 8 minutes on each side or until browned and caramelized. If you are using an indoor grill pan, you may need to cook them longer on each side. (The grill pan does not get as hot as an outdoor grill.) Allow the grilled pineapple to cool. When cool enough to handle, cut them into 1-inch chunks. Transfer them to a bowl.
3. Add the avocado to the pineapple along with the lime juice, jalapeño, salt and pepper, and cilantro; mix well to combine, and serve.

Olive Tapanade

Serves 12	

Carb Level: Low

Per serving:

Carbohydrate:	1.3 g
Protein:	0.0 g

This is a savory topping for Parmesan Crisps (see page 7). Great for olive lovers.

1 cup kalamata olives, pitted
2 cloves garlic
1 tablespoon lemon juice
¼ cup olive oil

½ teaspoon lemon zest
Freshly ground black pepper
to taste

Combine all the ingredients in a food processor; process until blended. Store refrigerated in airtight containers.

Mock Caviar

Serves 12	

Carb Level: Low

Per serving:

Carbohydrate:	4.4 g
Protein:	0.8 g

This is a great topping for Parmesan Crisps (see page 7) or cucumber slices.

2 eggplants, about 1 pound each
¼ cup olive oil
8 cloves garlic, skin on

3 tablespoons chopped parsley
Salt and freshly ground black
pepper to taste

1. Preheat oven to 425°.
2. Split the eggplants lengthwise and brush the cut surface with olive oil. Place on a baking sheet along with the whole garlic cloves. Bake for 30 to 40 minutes or until tender. Remove from oven and allow to cool.
3. Scoop out the flesh from the eggplant and transfer to the bowl of a food processor. Trim the root ends from the garlic cloves and squeeze out the garlic pulp; add the pulp to the eggplant. Add all the remaining ingredients and process until smooth. Store refrigerated in airtight containers.

Pesto Eggplant Caviar

1 large eggplant (1½ pounds)
1 red bell pepper, seeded,
  stemmed, and finely
  chopped
1 tablespoon olive oil
Salt
¼ cup pesto, homemade or
  prepared

1 large lemon
¼ cup fresh grated Parmesan
  cheese
Freshly ground black pepper
  to taste

Makes 1 ²/₃ cups
Carb Level: Moderate

Per serving:

Carbohydrate:	12.3 g
Protein:	5.4 g

This very versatile spread works great as a dip for vegetables or as a creative topping for roasted meats such as lamb.

1. Preheat oven to high broil.
2. Wash and dry the eggplant. Cut the eggplant in half and place on baking sheet cut-side down. Cook for a few minutes until the skin blisters and chars, checking several times and adjusting the position of the eggplant halves to make sure the skin cooks evenly. (This will impart a smoky flavor to the eggplant.)
3. Reduce oven temperature to 400°. Bake the eggplant for 50 minutes.
4. Meanwhile, sauté the red pepper in the olive oil over medium heat until tender; sprinkle with a pinch of salt and set aside.
5. Remove the eggplant from oven. Let cool for about 10 minutes. Scoop out the flesh and place in a food processor. Discard the remaining skin.
6. Add the pesto to the food processor. Use a citrus zester to get ½ teaspoon lemon zest; add to processor. Juice the lemon and add to the processor. Process the contents until fairly smooth.
7. Transfer to a bowl. Stir in the cooked red pepper and grated Parmesan cheese. Add salt and freshly ground black pepper to taste. Cover and refrigerate until cold.

Asian-Style Paste

Serves 12
Carb Level: Low

Per serving:	
Carbohydrate:	0.9 g
Protein:	1.3 g

Use this paste on top of sesame rice crackers for a flavorful pairing with an Asian-themed meal.

1 cup cream cheese
1 tablespoon wasabi
1 tablespoon grated gingerroot
1 tablespoon oyster sauce

2 tablespoons tamari sauce
Chili flakes to taste

Place all the ingredients in the bowl of a food processor; process until blended. Store refrigerated in airtight containers.

Jalapeño Paste

Serves 12
Carb Level: Low

Per serving:	
Carbohydrate:	2.3 g
Protein:	1.6 g

Use this paste on top of Spicy Jicama Chips (see page 5) for a flavorful pairing with a Mexican-themed meal.

6 jalapeños
2 tablespoons olive oil
1 cup cream cheese
2 tablespoons chopped cilantro leaves

1 teaspoon lime zest, finely grated
Salt and pepper to taste

1. Preheat oven to 400°.
2. Rub the jalapeños with olive oil and roast on a nonstick baking sheet for about 30 minutes, or until they turn dark brown. Transfer to a bowl and cover tightly with plastic wrap. Allow to sit for 15 minutes or until cool. Seed and skin the peppers. Mash the flesh together with the remaining ingredients in the bowl of a food processor; process until blended. Store refrigerated in airtight containers.

Sausage Appetizers

1 pound pork sausage meat
½ pound grated Cheddar
   cheese
4 ounces margarine, softened
6 ounces all-purpose flour

2 tablespoons paprika
Salt and freshly ground black
   pepper to taste

Serves 25
(makes 50 pieces)

Carb Level: Low

Per serving:	
Carbohydrate:	6.2 g
Protein:	6.0 g

These are savory little bites served hot from the oven—perfect for a cold-weather get-together.

ॐ

1. Preheat oven to 350°.
2. Form the sausage meat into fifty 1-inch balls. Place on a nonstick baking sheet and bake for 15 minutes. Transfer to paper towels to cool and drain.
3. Combine the remaining ingredients using the flat blade of an electric mixer. Wrap approximately 2 tablespoons of the dough around each sausage ball. Place the balls on an ungreased nonstick baking sheet and bake for 10 to 12 minutes, until golden. Spear with toothpicks and serve hot.

Food Safety

Food safety is based on the simple principle of "Hot Foods Hot—Cold Foods Cold". One of the best investments you can make is to have a quality freezer thermometer, refrigerator thermometer, and oven thermometer. Check them frequently to make sure your kitchen equipment is working properly.

Basic Party Dip
and Five Variations

4 ounces cream cheese, softened
12 ounces sour cream
Salt and freshly ground black pepper to taste

Mix together all the ingredients until smooth. Add the ingredients from one of the following variations. Keep tightly covered and refrigerated until ready to serve.

Blue Cheese Dip

1 recipe basic dip
4 ounces blue cheese, crumbled
1 tablespoon minced fresh onion
1 tablespoon lemon juice
½ cup buttermilk

This dip is great served with crackers, chips, or fresh vegetables.

Dill Dip

1 recipe basic dip
2 tablespoons dill weed
1 tablespoon minced fresh onion
1 tablespoon Beau Monde seasoning

This dip pairs well with fresh vegetables.

Serves 15

Carb Level: Low

Blue Cheese Dip

Per serving:

Carbohydrate:	1.9 g
Protein:	3.2 g

Dill Dip

Per serving:

Carbohydrate:	1.9 g
Protein:	3.0 g

Dips are an easy appetizer to prepare in advance—then just add to a garnished platter of chips or trimmed vegetables.

Basic Party Dip
and Five Variations (continued)

Seafood Dip

1 recipe basic dip
4 ounces cooked shrimp and crab, chopped
½ ounce dry onion soup mix
2 tablespoons chili sauce
1 tablespoon horseradish.

A delicious accompaniment with water crackers, jicama chips, or toasted party bread.

Creamy Onion Dip

1 recipe basic dip
1½ ounces dry onion soup mix
2 tablespoons snipped fresh chives.

This dip goes well with chips or fresh trimmed vegetables.

Picante Dip

1 recipe basic dip
6 ounces salsa
¼ cup fresh cilantro leaves, chopped
¼ cup stuffed olives, chopped

This dip is great with tortilla chips or fresh trimmed vegetables.

Serves 15	
Carb Level: Low	
Seafood Dip	
Per serving:	
Carbohydrate:	1.5 g
Protein:	1.4 g
Creamy Onion Dip	
Per serving:	
Carbohydrate:	3.2 g
Protein:	1.7 g
Picante Dip	
Per serving:	
Carbohydrate:	2.1 g
Protein:	1.5 g

Warm Spinach and Artichoke Dip

Serves 8
Carb Level: Moderate

Per serving:

Carbohydrate:	10.9 g
Protein:	5.4 g

Be sure to use plain, not marinated, canned artichoke hearts.

❧

2 tablespoons butter
1 cup sliced fresh mushrooms
1 small onion, chopped
¼ cup chopped yellow and/or red bell pepper
4 teaspoons all-purpose flour
⅛ teaspoon ground nutmeg
1 cup milk
1½ cups chopped fresh spinach
1 (14-ounce) can plain artichoke hearts, well drained and chopped
⅓ cup grated Parmesan or Romano cheese
1 tablespoon dry white wine
1 teaspoon Worcestershire sauce
Several dashes hot pepper sauce

1. Heat the butter in a medium-size sauté pan over medium heat. Cook the mushrooms, onion, and peppers until they are tender. Stir in the flour and nutmeg. Add the milk all at once. Cook, stirring continually, over medium heat until thick and bubbly.

2. Stir in the remaining ingredients; cook, stirring, until heated through. Transfer to a soufflé dish and serve immediately. You can refrigerate the dip and when you are ready to serve; reheat in a 400° oven for about 20 minutes or until bubbly.

CHAPTER 2

Five or Fewer Ingredients

Asian Salmon	18
Steamed Clams with Cilantro-Garlic Essence ❖	19
Chipotle Shrimp ❖	20
Creamy Garlic and Fennel Soup ❖	21
Peppered Swordfish ❖	22
Roasted Chicken Stuffed with Herbed Goat Cheese	23
Balsamic-Marinated Beef Tenderloin ❖	24
Roasted Tomato Onion Soup	25
Sage- and Pancetta-Wrapped Shrimp	26
Smoked Trout and Watercress Salad ❖	27
Spanish Stuffed Veal Chops ❖	28
Tuna Steaks with Wasabi-Coconut Sauce ❖	29
Wine and Cheese Fondue	30
Lemon-Spiked Pineapple Smoothie ❖	31
Pineapple-Ginger Smoothie ❖	32

❖ **Indicates Easy Recipe** ❖

Asian Salmon

4 (6-ounce) center-cut salmon
   fillets, skin on
½ cup teriyaki sauce
3 bunches scallions

Freshly cracked black pepper
Salt to taste

Serves 4
Carb Level: Low

Per serving:

Carbohydrate:	9.6 g
Protein:	38.5 g

Use the freshest salmon available and a low-sodium teriyaki sauce to get the best flavors.

                  ॐ

1. Remove any bones from the salmon. Place the salmon in shallow casserole dish. Cover with teriyaki sauce and allow to marinate in the refrigerator for 5 to 10 minutes.
2. Rinse the scallions and trim off and discard the root ends. Reserve 6 scallions. Split the remaining scallions in half, lengthwise, and trim off and discard all but 1 inch of the green tops. Cut the scallions into 1-inch pieces. Place the trimmed scallions in a nonstick skillet, uncovered, with enough salted water to cover. Bring to a boil, then lower heat and cook, uncovered, until the scallions are soft, about 3 to 5 minutes. Drain and keep warm.
3. Remove the salmon from the marinade and reserve the marinade. Press ½ teaspoon of the coarsely ground black pepper into the skinless side of each salmon fillet. Heat 1 very large nonstick skillet or 2 smaller ones until almost smoking. Cook the fillets skin side up and uncovered over medium-high heat for 3 minutes. Turn over and cook for another 3 minutes, or until the skin is golden brown and crispy, then turn to very low heat.
4. While the salmon is cooking on low, finely dice the remaining scallions and add them to the reserved marinade. Add the marinade and ¼ cup water to the pan(s) with the salmon. Bring to a simmer and cook, uncovered, until the salmon has reached serving temperature. Season with salt and pepper to taste. Serve immediately with the boiled scallions.

Steamed Clams
with Cilantro-Garlic Essence

4 dozen littleneck clams
½ cup unsalted whipped
   butter, well chilled and
   cut into pieces
½ teaspoon whole black
   peppercorns
1 teaspoon salt

1 cup coarsely chopped
   cilantro leaves, plus extra,
   finely chopped, for garnish
1 clove garlic, minced

Serves 4
Carb Level: Low

Per serving:

Carbohydrate:	2.3 g
Protein:	2.6 g

Be sure you put an empty bowl on the table for the shells.

෴

1. Scrub the clams well under cold running water. Discard any clams with open or partially open shells. Place the clams in a large heavy pot along with ½ cup water and all the remaining ingredients.
2. Bring the mixture to a boil. Cover the pot with a tight-fitted lid and cook over high heat for 6 to 8 minutes, shaking the pot back and forth every so often to cook the clams evenly. Remove from heat when the clam shells open up.
3. Transfer the clams to 4 large, flat soup plates and pour the broth over them. Garnish with the finely chopped cilantro. Serve immediately.

Clam Facts

When buying hard-shell clams in the shell, make sure the shells are tightly closed. If the shell is open slightly, tap it to see if it snaps shut. If the shell does not close tightly, discard the clam. Cook clams gently to prevent toughening the meat.

Chipotle Shrimp

1 pound (about 32) uncooked
  medium shrimp
6 tablespoons unsalted butter
2 heaping tablespoons chopped
  canned chipotle peppers in
  adobo sauce

1 small bunch cilantro, chopped
Salt and freshly ground black
  pepper to taste

Makes about 32 pieces

Carb Level: Low

Per serving:

Carbohydrate:	0.4 g
Protein:	6.2 g

Chipotle peppers are actually dried smoked jalapeños. You can find them in the Hispanic food section of your supermarket.

1. Clean and devein the shrimp, leaving the tails on if possible.
2. Melt the butter in a 12-inch nonstick skillet over medium heat. When the butter is bubbling and starting to foam, add the chipotle peppers and shrimp, and increase heat to high.
3. Stirring constantly, cook the shrimp until just firm, no more than 4 minutes. Do not overcook. Sprinkle with cilantro and salt, and toss.
4. Put the shrimp and sauce on individual plates or a platter and serve hot.

Unsalted Butter

Unsalted butter is sometimes referred to as sweet butter. Many cooks prefer it because it does not contain any salt at all. It is more perishable than salted butter because it does not contain any preservatives, and it should be stored in the freezer if you are not using it right away. Butter can be frozen for up to 6 months.

Creamy Garlic and Fennel Soup

14–16 cloves garlic, peeled and
   trimmed
2 cups heavy cream
2 large fennel bulbs
   (1 pound each)

1 teaspoon salt
Finely ground white pepper

> **Serves 6–8**
> (makes about 8 cups)
>
> **Carb Level: Low**
>
> Per serving:
>
> | | |
> |---|---|
> | Carbohydrate: | 6.2 g |
> | Protein: | 2.0 g |
>
> This is a great do-ahead recipe—refrigerate until ready to reheat and serve.
>
> ❧

1. Place the garlic and cream in a medium-size pot with a cover and bring to a light boil over medium heat. Lower heat, cover, and gently simmer for 30 to 40 minutes, until the garlic cloves are very soft.
2. Trim and clean the fennel by cutting off the stalks and wispy sprigs (fronds) from the bulbs and reserve for later use. Cut the bulb in half lengthwise and use a small, sharp knife to trim out the root. Keep the fronds refrigerated, wrapped in a very moist paper towel. Keep the stalks and bulb portion and discard the root trimmings.
3. Cut the bulb portion and the darker stalks into ½-inch pieces. Place in colander and wash thoroughly to remove any dirt. Drain well.
4. Add the fennel and 3 cups of water to the garlic-cream mixture. Bring just to a boil, lower heat, and cover. Simmer for another 40 minutes, until the fennel is very soft.
5. Transfer to blender or food processor and purée in several batches until very smooth (doing so carefully, because the mixture is very hot). Return to the pot and add the salt and white pepper to taste. Heat for several minutes until the soup thickens up a bit; adjust seasoning to taste.
6. Finely chop the fennel fronds and scatter over the soup for garnish. Serve hot, or keep refrigerated and gently reheat before serving.

ℰ Buying Garlic

Most supermarket produce sections carry fresh garlic already cleaned, in jars or plastic containers. Older garlic cloves will appear wrinkled and spotted and are bitter. Make sure the cloves have an unblemished, even ivory color, which indicates freshness.

Peppered Swordfish

Serves 4

Carb Level: Low

Per serving:

Carbohydrate:	3.0 g
Protein:	34.1 g

The flesh of the steaks should be gleaming and bright. Spotting, browning, or any discoloration indicates fish that is aging.

∾

4 (6-½ ounce) swordfish steaks
¼ cup extra-virgin olive oil
Salt and freshly ground black
   pepper

2 medium-size red and
2 medium-size yellow bell
   peppers

1. Lightly brush each side of the steaks with some of the olive oil, seasoned lightly with salt and freshly cracked black pepper. Sprinkle a little bit of salt on each side of the swordfish steaks. Refrigerate while preparing the bell peppers.
2. Cut the peppers in half, discarding the stems, seeds, and whitish inner membrane. Cut the peppers into long, thin strips, no more than ¼ inch wide and about 1½ to 2 inches long.
3. Heat the remaining oil in a large heavy nonstick skillet on medium-high heat. Add the peppers, about ½ teaspoon black pepper, and ½ teaspoon salt. Cook uncovered, stirring occasionally, until the peppers are soft and lightly browned, about 20 minutes. Set the peppers aside and keep warm.
4. Heat the same skillet until very hot, almost smoking. Add the swordfish and cook over medium-high heat so that the fish is browned on the outside but moist on the inside, about 4 minutes per side; turn the steaks once through the cooking process. (Check for doneness by cutting into the center of the steaks with a thin-bladed knife: the flesh should be flaky with no translucence remaining.) Heat the bell peppers if necessary and serve on top of the steaks. Garnish with more freshly ground black pepper if desired.

What Are Capers?

Capers are the flower bud of a bush that is native to the Mediterranean and parts of Asia. Capers range in size from tiny, known as the nonpareil variety from southern France, to the Italian caper which is as large as the tip of you little finger. Capers are generally packed in brine and should be rinsed before using. They are a flavorful addition to many sauces and condiments.

Roasted Chicken Stuffed with Herbed Goat Cheese

3 packed cups fresh basil leaves
(about 2 large bunches)
8 ounces fresh goat cheese,
preferably flavored with garlic
and herbs, well chilled

2 tablespoons butter
Freshly ground black pepper and
salt to taste
5-pound roasting chicken

Serves 6
Carb Level: Low

Per serving:	
Carbohydrate:	0.9 g
Protein:	52.4 g

The roasted chicken can be prepared a day in advance. Refrigerate and just warm lightly before serving.

1. Preheat oven to 350°.
2. Rinse the basil leaves and pat dry with paper towels. In a food processor, combine the basil, goat cheese, and freshly ground black pepper; process until the basil is incorporated and the cheese is smooth (the mixture may turn a pale green); set aside.
3. Make sure the giblets are removed from the inside cavity of the chicken. Rinse the chicken, inside and out, and pat dry with paper towels. Using poultry shears, cut off the wing tips of the chicken. Starting at the neck of the chicken, slip your fingers under the skin of the breast, carefully separating the skin from the flesh. Continue downward and, with your index finger, separate the skin around the thighs.
4. Using your fingers or a spoon, push the cheese mixture under the skin to cover the entire breasts and thighs as evenly as possible (press on the skin to distribute evenly). You will have a layer of cheese approximately ¼-inch thick under the skin.
5. Rub the outside of the chicken with butter. Sprinkle the entire chicken, including the internal cavity, with salt and freshly ground black pepper. Truss the chicken by tying the legs together with a 6- to 8-inch piece of butcher's twine. Roast on a rack in a heavy, shallow baking pan, uncovered, for about 1½ hours or until a meat thermometer inserted into a thigh reads 160°. Check on the chicken every 30 minutes during the roasting time and baste with pan juices. (Make a tent with tin foil to cover the chicken if the skin becomes too brown before the proper internal temperature is achieved.)
6. Remove from oven and let rest for about 10 minutes. Carve as desired, but it is best if cut into quarters, with the backbone removed.

Balsamic-Marinated Beef Tenderloin

Serves 6
Carb Level: Low
Per serving:
Carbohydrate: 2.0 g
Protein: 40.3 g

This delicious recipe is also great on the grill. Any extra balsamic glaze also works well on roasted vegetables.

∿

6 (10-ounce) 1-inch-thick beef
  tenderloin fillets
½ cup extra-virgin olive oil,
  plus extra for grilling
½ cup, plus 2 tablespoons
  balsamic vinegar

2 tablespoons very finely
  chopped fresh rosemary
Salt and coarsely ground black
  pepper

1. Place the meat in a shallow casserole dish. Mix together the olive oil, the 2 tablespoons of balsamic vinegar, and the rosemary in a small bowl; pour over the fillets, turning the meat to ensure the steaks are evenly coated. Let marinate in the refrigerator, covered, for 2 hours, turning the fillets after 1 hour.
2. Remove the fillets from the marinade. Sprinkle salt and pepper on both sides.
3. Coat a grill pan or sauté pan lightly with oil. Preheat the pan until very hot, almost smoking, and cook the fillets for about 3 to 4 minutes on each side for medium-rare. (Increase cooking time by 2-minute increments per side for each of medium, medium-well, and well-done.)
4. Place the remaining balsamic vinegar in small saucepan and cook over medium heat until reduced to about half (¼ cup).
5. Let the fillets sit for a few minutes after they are done cooking, then drizzle with a little of the reduced balsamic vinegar; serve immediately.

Olive Oil

The difference between extra-virgin olive oil and other types of olive oil is mostly in the taste. Extra-virgin olive oil is from the first pressing of the olives. It is fruitier and more intense in flavor than other olive oils. It is best in vinaigrettes, chilled soups, or drizzled over any dish. Other olive oils are usually better to cook with because they have a higher smoking point.

Roasted Tomato Onion Soup

4 large ripe tomatoes (about 2
   pounds total)
8 medium onions (about 2
   pounds total), unpeeled
5 tablespoons extra-virgin olive
   oil, divided, plus extra for
   garnish

½–⅔ cup water
½ cup heavy cream
Salt and freshly ground black
   pepper to taste

Serves 6
(makes about 5 cups)

Carb Level: Moderate

Per serving:

Carbohydrate:	19.2 g
Protein:	3.2 g

Use fresh tomatoes
from the farmers'
market, if possible,
for the best flavor.

❧

1. Preheat oven to 250°. Bring a large pot of water to a boil. Fill a medium-sized bowl ¾ full with cold water and ice; have it ready next to the stovetop.
2. To skin the tomatoes, make a small **X** in the bottom of each tomato using a small, sharp knife and cut out the core, keeping the tomato whole. Plunge the tomatoes in the boiling water for 1 minute. Using tongs, remove the tomatoes from the boiling water and drop them into the bowl of ice water; let them sit for a couple of minutes. (This process is called *shocking*. It stops the tomatoes from cooking any further.) Drain the tomatoes and peel off the skin using a small paring knife (it should come off very easily).
3. Cut the tomatoes in half and place cut-side down on a large baking sheet. Place the whole, unpeeled onions on the baking sheet with the tomatoes. Drizzle 2 tablespoons of the olive oil over the tomatoes and onions, using your hands to coat them well. Sprinkle the tomatoes with salt. Roast for 3 hours.
4. Remove the skins from the onions and place 5 of them in a food processor along with the tomatoes; process until very smooth. Add ½ to ⅔ cup water and the remaining 3 tablespoons of olive oil, and process again.
5. Transfer to a bowl and slowly add cream, stirring well to mix. Add salt and freshly ground black pepper to taste. Cut up the remaining peeled onions and spoon them over the top of the soup along with a drizzle of olive oil for garnish. Serve hot or at room temperature. (If not serving right away, you may need to add more water, as the soup will thicken.)

Sage- and Pancetta-Wrapped Shrimp

Serves 4
Carb Level: Low

Per serving:

Carbohydrate:	1.7 g
Protein:	46.4 g

Pancetta is a cured Italian bacon that is not smoked. It is available from Italian specialty stores.

∾

1½ pounds uncooked large shrimp (about 20 total)
6 ounces thinly sliced pancetta (10 slices)
28 fresh sage leaves (about 2 bunches)
⅓ cup sherry vinegar or cider vinegar

1. Remove the shells and tails from the shrimp. Devein the shrimp. Cut the slices of pancetta in half. Tear the sage leaves from the stems.
2. On a flat surface, lay out a half slice of pancetta. Place 1 large or 2 small leaves of sage on top, then place 1 shrimp across the pancetta and sage. Roll the pancetta around the shrimp and secure it closed with a toothpick (exposing the tail and head ends of the shrimp). Repeat with the rest of the shrimp.
3. Heat a medium-size nonstick skillet on medium-high flame. Place half of the rolled shrimp in the pan (the pancetta should sizzle). Cook until the pancetta is light brown and crispy on each side. Place the shrimp on paper towels to drain, and cover to keep warm. Repeat for the second half of rolled shrimp.
4. Immediately after all the shrimp has been cooked, keeping the pan on the flame, pour in the sherry vinegar and cook down to a syrup-like consistency. Place the shrimp on a platter and pour the hot reduced vinegar over the shrimp. Serve immediately.

When Is a Shrimp a Jumbo?

Shrimp is sold in the following categories:

Colossal	*less than 10 pieces per pound*
Jumbo	*11–15 pieces per pound*
Extra-large	*16–20 pieces per pound*
Large	*21–30 pieces per pound*
Medium	*31–35 pieces per pound*
Small	*36–45 pieces per pound*
Miniature	*100 pieces per pound*

Smoked Trout and Watercress Salad

*6 small smoked trout fillets
(about 5–6 inches in length)*
*3 large bunches fresh
watercress*

Salt
6 tablespoons walnut oil
Freshly ground black pepper

1. Carefully the remove skin, if any, from the trout fillets. Cut each fillet in half lengthwise; set aside. Wash the watercress and pat dry in paper towels. Trim off all but 1 inch of the stem.
2. Bring 3 cups of water and ¼ teaspoon salt to a boil. Add half the watercress. Cook for 1 minute. Reserving ⅔ cup of the cooking liquid, drain immediately in a colander under cold running water
3. Place the cooked watercress in the bowl of food processor and process slowly, adding (at a drizzle) the warm cooking water only until you have a thick paste. With the processor running, slowly add 4 tablespoons of the walnut oil. The dressing should be smooth and fairly thick. Add salt and freshly ground black pepper to taste. You will have about ¾ cup dressing.
4. To assemble the salads, portion the remaining fresh watercress in the center of 6 large chilled plates. Drizzle a little dressing over the watercress. Place 2 smoked trout pieces, crisscrossed, on top of the watercress. Drizzle the remaining dressing around the salad and across the center of the trout. You can also serve the salad on a large platter and arrange the trout fillets in a star shape.

Simple Success with a Few Ingredients

Quality ingredients are the key to success with recipes that use only a few items. Buy fruit at the peak of ripeness, use only the freshest fish, and choose high-quality cheeses. You won't be disappointed.

Serves 6
Carb Level: Low

Per serving:

Carbohydrate:	0.2 g
Protein:	16.8 g

Smoked trout is available in the refrigerated section at better fish and seafood counters.

〜

Spanish Stuffed Veal Chops

Serves 4
Carb Level: Low

Per serving:	
Carbohydrate:	0.7 g
Protein:	37.3 g

This is also a great grilling recipe. Using a toothpick to secure the filling makes the chops easier to turn while cooking.

∽

4 (10-ounce) 1-inch-thick veal rib chops
Salt and freshly ground black pepper to taste
8 ounces Manchego cheese
½ cup coarsely chopped pimento-stuffed green olives (3-ounce jar, drained)
1 bunch chervil, leaves chopped

1. Preheat broiler. With a sharp knife, cut a 2-inch-wide horizontal pocket in the side of each chop. The pocket should be about 1½ to 2 inches deep. Season the chops lightly on each side with salt and freshly ground black pepper.
2. Remove the rind from the cheese and discard. Cut the cheese into ¼-inch cubes. Place the cheese, olives, and chervil in a bowl and lightly season with salt and freshly ground black pepper; toss until evenly mixed.
3. Stuff each chop with about a quarter of the cheese mixture. Secure closed with a toothpick if necessary. Broil for about 3 minutes per side for medium-rare. (Increase cooking time by 2-minute increments per side for each of medium, medium-well, and well-done.) Serve immediately. Top with any remaining cheese and olive mixture.

The Vegetable Everyone Loves to Hate

Brussels Sprouts—⅓-cup serving contains 2.6 grams of carbohydrates. Brussels sprouts are believed to have been cultivated in sixteenth-century Belgium. It is best to store unwashed sprouts in an airtight container for up to 3 days—any longer and a strong undesirable flavor will develop. Brussels sprouts are a cruciferous vegetable, high in vitamins A and C and a good source of iron.

Tuna Steaks
with Wasabi-Coconut Sauce

1 (13½-ounce) can unsweetened
  coconut milk
1 tablespoon wasabi powder
Salt

6 (5-ounce) 1-inch-thick tuna
  steaks (ahi or yellowtail
  sushi grade)
Freshly ground black pepper

1. Mix together the coconut milk and wasabi powder in saucepan using a wire whisk until the wasabi is thoroughly dissolved. Let stand at room temperature for 30 minutes.
2. Bring the coconut-wasabi mixture to a simmer, whisking constantly. Lower heat to medium and reduce mixture to 1½ cups. This will take approximately 5 minutes. Add ½ teaspoon salt and stir. Remove from heat.
3. Season each side of the tuna steaks with salt and freshly ground black pepper. Place 2 large nonstick skillets over high heat. When very hot, almost smoking, add the tuna steaks. Cook for 2 minutes and turn. Cook for 1 to 2 minutes more, until the tuna is seared on the outside but still rare on the inside.
4. Remove the tuna from the skillets and let sit for 1 minute. Reheat the coconut-wasabi sauce gently over low heat. Cut the tuna on the bias into ½-inch-thick slices, pour the sauce over the fish, and serve immediately.

Serves 6
Carb Level: Low

Per serving:

Carbohydrate:	2.5 g
Protein:	40.6 g

This sauce has a kick—you may want to serve it on the side if you don't know the tastes of your dining guests.

℘

Wine and Cheese Fondue

Serves 6
Carb Level: Low

Per serving:

Carbohydrate:	3.5 g
Protein:	45.5 g

This is a great savory fondue. Use a good-quality wine to enhance the flavor of the Gruyère cheese.

∾

2 pounds Gruyère cheese
3 tablespoons all-purpose flour, divided
2 cups chardonnay or other dry white wine

Salt
Freshly ground white pepper

1. Using a sharp knife, remove the rind, if any, from the cheese. Grate the cheese using the large holes of a box grater. Mix with 1½ tablespoons of the flour.
2. Place the floured cheese in a medium-size heavy saucepan (or fondue pot). Add the wine and ½ teaspoon salt, and bring to a simmer, stirring frequently. Lower heat to medium and stir vigorously with a wooden spoon until the cheese is completely melted, about 5 minutes. Add the remaining flour, stirring constantly. Cook for about 2 minutes, until the floury, starchy taste is gone.
3. The sauce should be smooth, thick, and creamy. If it is too thick, add more wine that has been warmed first. Adjust seasoning to taste. Serve with fresh strawberries and grapes, vegetables, or cooked chicken breast strips.

ℰ Ahi Tuna Steaks

When using ahi tuna steaks as a grilled entrée, consider grilling an extra steak and make your own grilled tuna salad. Season and cook the tuna steak until just done throughout, but not dried out. Allow to cool, wrap tightly, and refrigerate. To make the salad, lightly flake the tuna and mix with your favorite dressing. You can make a mesquite-flavored tuna salad by using a dry spice rub on the tuna before grilling. Experiment and add different flavoring ingredients such as capers, fresh dill, chopped chives, or minced scallions.

Lemon-Spiked Pineapple Smoothie

1 medium-size ripe pineapple
6 tablespoons freshly squeezed
*   lemon juice, plus thinly*
*   sliced lemons for garnish*

Packets of sugar substitute
*   (optional)*

Serves 6
Carb Level: Moderate

Per serving:	
Carbohydrate:	13.1 g
Protein:	0.4 g

You can buy fresh pineapples already trimmed at larger supermarkets. Remember to check the freshness date when using this time-saving step.

1. Peel the pineapple and cut out the core. Cut the fruit into small pieces. Place in food processor and process to a somewhat smooth pulpy consistency. Transfer to a large pitcher.
2. Add the lemon juice, 4 cups of cold water, and 3 packets at a time of sugar substitute to the desired sweetness, stirring until dissolved. Chill for several hours and serve in glasses over ice with a thin slice of lemon for garnish.

Just Plain Nuts

Toasted chopped nuts are always a nice addition to simple poultry and fish dishes. Here are the carb and protein counts per ¼ cup for some of our favorite nuts:

	Carbohydrate	*Protein*
Almonds	*7.2 g*	*7.1 g*
Walnuts	*3.8 g*	*7.6 g*
Peanuts	*5.9 g*	*9.4 g*
Cashews	*9.2 g*	*5.3 g*
Pecans	*4.9 g*	*2.1 g*
Macadamia nuts	*4.6 g*	*2.8 g*

Pineapple-Ginger Smoothie

Serves 2

Carb Level: Moderate

Per serving:

| Carbohydrate: | 19.3 g |
| Protein: | 4.0 g |

This is a refreshing drink for an outdoor dinner. Using wineglasses "dresses up" this nonalcoholic cocktail.

1 cup unsweetened pineapple
  juice
½ cup plain yogurt
3 tablespoons grated fresh
  ginger

6–8 ice cubes
Ground cinnamon or ground
  nutmeg for garnish

Put all the ingredients, except the garnish, in a blender; process on high until smooth and creamy and all ice particles have disappeared. Add sugar substitute if desired. Serve immediately in chilled wineglasses. Sprinkle a little ground cinnamon or ground nutmeg on top for added spice.

Summer Berries

Use fresh berries when in season for smoothies. Half of a cup of fresh strawberries contains 5.25 grams of carbs and a great flavor punch.

CHAPTER 3

French Entrées

Pork and Veal Pâté ❖	34
Crêpes ❖	35
Crêpe Fillings	36
Braised Dover Sole with Béchamel and Vegetables	38
Mustard-Glazed Monkfish Wrapped in Bacon	40
Chicken Breasts Chasseur	41
Red Snapper with Cayenne Tomato Sauce ❖	42
Roasted Duck with Lemon	43
Grilled Lamb Chops with Provençal Roasted Tomatoes ❖	44
Baked Haddock with Parsley and Lemon	46
Halibut with Porcinis, Shallots, and Tomatoes	47
Lemon Chicken	48
Beef Provençal ❖	49
Trout Grenobloise ❖	50
Veal Stew Blanquette	51

❖ **Indicates Easy Recipe** ❖

Pork and Veal Pâté

Serves 6
Carb Level: Low

Per serving:

Carbohydrate:	2.4 g
Protein:	19.7 g

A French classic, this pâté has a crumbly mixture because it is not weighted during the cooling and setting process.

∿

1¼ pounds pork shoulder or rump, cut into 1-inch cubes
½ pound veal shoulder, cut into 1-inch cubes
1 small yellow onion, peeled and chopped
½ pound salt pork, finely chopped

¼ teaspoon ground cloves
¼ teaspoon ground cinnamon
Salt and freshly ground black pepper

1. With a sharp knife, finely chop the pork and veal to the texture of ground meat.
2. Put the chopped meat, onions, and 1½ cups water in a large pot; cook over medium heat until the liquid has evaporated and meat begins to brown, about 30 minutes.
3. Put the salt pork into a small saucepan; cook uncovered over medium heat, stirring often, until the fat has been rendered and the pork is golden brown, about 30 minutes.
4. Add the salt pork and the rendered fat to the meat mixture along with the remaining ingredients. Transfer to a container with a cover and set aside to let cool to room temperature. Cover and refrigerate for a least 2 hours before serving.

The Sophisticated Flavor of Shallots

Shallots are favored for their mild onion flavor and are used in the same manner as onions. Shallots are used as a staple in French classic sauces and dressings. Two tablespoons of shallots contain 3.4 grams of carbohydrate. Two tablespoons of onions contains 1.7 grams of carbohydrate. Shallots are used in much smaller quantities than onions and have a much bolder flavor. Consider substituting small amounts of sautéed shallots in place of a larger quantity of onions for a more sophisticated flavor.

Crêpes

2 large eggs
1 cup milk
1/3 cup water
1 cup flour

1/4 teaspoon salt
2 tablespoons melted butter,
    plus 2 teaspoons butter for
    coating

1. Place the eggs, milk, water, flour, salt, and 2 tablespoons of melted butter in a blender and process until smooth.
2. Heat a nonstick 6- or 7-inch crêpe pan over medium-high heat. Coat the pan lightly with butter. Lift the pan from the heat and pour in 2 or 3 tablespoons of batter, tilting and rotating the pan to coat the surface. Cook until almost dry on top and lightly browned around the edges. Loosen the edges with a rubber spatula and flip the crêpe over using your fingers or the spatula. Cook the other side for about 15 seconds. Turn the crêpe out onto a paper towel to cool and repeat with the remaining batter. You may need to add more butter to the pan.
3. After cooling, store between layers of waxed paper. If serving immediately, cover the crêpes with foil to keep warm in a 200° oven.

Serves 10	
Carb Level: Moderate	
Per serving:	
Carbohydrate:	10.8 g
Protein:	3.4 g

An all-time favorite. Versatility is the key: great for breakfast, lunch, or dinner at any time of year.

Crêpes

Crêpes originated in Brittany, in the northwestern section of France. Crêpe is French for "pancake." Crêpes can be folded into various shapes for decorative presentation. Roll and slice them for attractive pinwheels for appetizers using the smoked salmon filling, or place the filling in the center and fold in the edges on four sides for an open-face look. Or—you can always use the traditional "roll 'em up" style for ease and simplicity.

Crêpe Fillings

Sausage and Cheese Filling

1 pound spicy Italian sausage
1 cup ricotta cheese
½ cup grated Parmesan cheese
2 cloves garlic, minced

Salt and freshly ground black
* pepper*
Fresh chopped parsley
* (optional)*

1. Heat a nonstick sauté pan over medium heat. Add the sausage and cook until lightly browned. Stir throughout the cooking process to break up the sausage into small pieces. Remove with a slotted spoon and transfer to a small mixing bowl. Add the remaining ingredients, mix well, and adjust seasoning as desired.
2. Preheat oven to 325°.
3. Spoon about ⅓ to ½ cup of filling in a ribbon down the center of each crêpe and roll up. Arrange in a lightly oiled baking dish. Bake, partially covered, for about 15 to 18 minutes, until heated through. Garnish with parsley if desired and serve immediately.

Smoked Salmon and Ricotta Cheese Filling

2 tablespoons chopped fresh dill
¾ cup ricotta cheese
8 ounces cream cheese, soft-
* ened at room temperature*
2 tablespoons minced red onion

8 ounces smoked salmon
Salt and freshly ground black
* pepper*

1. Mix together all the ingredients in a bowl.
2. Spoon about ⅓ to ½ cup of filling in a ribbon down the center of each crêpe and roll up. Serve at room temperature. Slice into pinwheels for a great appetizer.

**Sausage
and Cheese Filling
Serves 6**

Carb Level: Low

Per serving:

Carbohydrate:	2.7 g
Protein:	16.3 g

**Smoked Salmon and
Ricotta Cheese Filling
Serves 6**

Carb Level: Low

Per serving:

Carbohydrate:	3.0 g
Protein:	13.5 g

(recipe continues on the next page)

Crêpe Fillings (continued)

Three-Cheese Filling

2 eggs
¾ cup Gruyère cheese, grated
1 cup ricotta cheese
¾ cup goat cheese
⅛ teaspoon freshly ground nutmeg

Salt and freshly ground black
   pepper
Chopped fresh herbs for garnish
   (optional)

1. Beat the eggs in a medium-size mixing bowl. Add the remaining ingredients and mix well.
2. Preheat oven to 325°.
3. Spoon about ⅓ to ½ cup of filling in a ribbon down the center of each crêpe and roll up. Arrange in a lightly oiled baking dish. Bake, partially covered, for about 18 to 22 minutes, until the filling is cooked and heated through. Note that there is raw egg in the filling and you will want to actually "cook" the filling. Garnish with chopped herbs, if desired, and serve immediately.

Three-Cheese Filling Serves 6	
Carb Level: Low	
Per serving:	
Carbohydrate:	2.7 g
Protein:	17.3 g
❧	

Ham and Asparagus Filling

1½ cups ricotta cheese
½ cup grated Parmesan cheese
2 teaspoons chopped fresh
   tarragon
8 ounces deli-sliced ham, chopped

1½ pounds asparagus spears,
   cleaned and cooked
Salt and freshly ground black
   pepper

1. Mix together the ricotta, Parmesan, tarragon, and ham in a medium-size mixing bowl until thoroughly combined.
2. Preheat oven to 325°.
3. Spoon about ⅓ to ½ cup of filling in a ribbon down the center of each crêpe. Top the filling with asparagus spears, with the tips just poking out of the ends. Roll up each crêpe and arrange in a lightly oiled baking dish. Bake, partially covered, for about 15 to 18 minutes, until heated through. Serve immediately.

Ham and Asparagus Filling Serves 6	
Carb Level: Low	
Per serving:	
Carbohydrate:	4.6 g
Protein:	11.0 g
❧	

Braised Dover Sole
with Béchamel and Vegetables

Serves 4
Carb Level: Moderate

Per serving:	
Carbohydrate:	17.9 g
Protein:	19.4 g

This is a beautiful presentation, worth the effort for an intimate dining setting with close friends.

∽

1 teaspoon canola oil
1½ teaspoons unsalted butter,
    softened, divided
1 carrot, julienned
2 ribs celery, julienned
1 leek, white part only,
    washed well and julienned
Salt and freshly ground white
    pepper
1 tablespoon minced shallots
4 (6-ounce) Dover sole fillets

1 cup dry white wine
½ cup chicken stock
1 recipe béchamel sauce
    (see following)
Juice of ½ lemon
1 tablespoon chopped fresh
    flat-leaf parsley for garnish

1. Heat a large nonstick sauté pan over medium heat. Combine the oil and 1 teaspoon of the butter and heat until it starts to foam. Add the carrot, celery, and leek. Sauté until just tender, remove from heat, and set aside. Season with salt and pepper.

2. Preheat the oven to 325°. Using the rest of the butter, lightly brush the bottom of an ovenproof pan large enough to hold all of the fish. Sprinkle the shallots on the bottom of the pan. Season both sides of the sole with salt and pepper. Place the fillets on top of the shallots and add the wine and chicken stock.

3. Place the pan over high heat on the stovetop, uncovered, until the stock is simmering. Cover the pan with foil and transfer it to the oven for about 15 minutes or until the fillets have cooked through. To check the fish for doneness, use a thin-bladed knife and poke into the center of the thickest part of the fillet. The flesh should be firm and flaky with no translucence.

(recipe continues on the next page)

Braised Dover Sole
with Béchamel and Vegetables (continued)

4. Using a long, slotted spatula, carefully lift the fillets from the pan and set aside. Strain the pan juices through a fine-mesh sieve into a medium-sized saucepan. Return the fillets to the pan and cover to keep warm. (Move the fish carefully, as the fillets will break apart if handled too roughly.)

5. Add the béchamel sauce to the saucepan and cook over medium heat. Whisk constantly for about 5 minutes or until the sauce has thickened. Whisk in the lemon juice and season with salt and pepper. Fold in the reserved vegetables and bring to a simmer.

6. Place each Dover sole fillet in the center of a plate and pour the sauce and vegetables around the fish. Garnish with chopped parsley.

Béchamel Sauce

1½ tablespoons cornstarch
1½ cups milk
3 whole cloves
½ small onion
1 bay leaf
Salt and freshly ground white pepper

1. Place the cornstarch in a heavy-bottomed saucepan. Whisk in ½ cup of milk until very smooth. Whisk in the remaining milk. Stick the cloves in the onion and add to the saucepan along with the bay leaf.

2. Cook over low heat, uncovered and stirring frequently, for about 12 to 15 minutes, until the mixture is hot and well infused with the flavors of the onion, clove, and bay leaf. The sauce should be fragrant. Increase the heat and simmer, stirring constantly, for about 5 minutes until it thickens. Strain and adjust seasoning to taste.

Mustard-Glazed Monkfish Wrapped in Bacon

Serves 6
Carb Level: Low

Per serving:

Carbohydrate:	2.1 g
Protein:	17.6 g

You'll consider this a very easy recipe to prepare the second time—and this one is a sure repeat.

❧

12 slices apple-wood-smoked or other good-quality bacon
6 (6-ounce) monkfish fillets
⅔ cup Dijon mustard
Salt and freshly ground black pepper
2 tablespoons tarragon

1. Preheat oven to 350°.
2. Place the bacon on a nonstick baking sheet and precook for about 8 minutes. The bacon should be almost fully cooked but still pliable. Drain the bacon on paper towels; discard the fat from the baking sheet.
3. Make sure the monkfish is trimmed of all membranes and dark spots. Season the monkfish with salt and pepper. Rub each fillet with 2 tablespoons of the mustard to coat completely.
4. Wrap each fillet with 2 slices of bacon, making sure the bacon doesn't overlap. Secure the bacon with toothpicks if necessary. Wrap each fillet tightly in plastic wrap, twisting the ends closed, and refrigerate for about 1 hour.
5. Preheat the oven to 375°.
6. Unwrap the fish and place on an oiled baking sheet. Bake for about 20 to 25 minutes until the fish is almost cooked. Increase the oven temperature to low broil. To finish, place the fish under the broiler for just about 30 seconds to crisp the bacon.
7. Drizzle a bit of the natural pan juices over the fish and sprinkle with chopped tarragon. Serve immediately.

Poor Man's Lobster?

Monkfish has been described as the poor man's lobster even though it has no resemblance to lobster whatsoever. Cooked properly, it has the texture of shellfish and does not have the "flakiness" of most fish. Mild in flavor and moderately firm in texture, it is a hearty fish.

Chicken Breasts Chasseur

4 (6-ounce) bone-in chicken
   breasts with skin
Salt and freshly ground black
   pepper
2 teaspoons olive oil, divided
1 medium carrot, chopped
½ cup chopped onion

2 cups beef broth
2 cups sliced button mushrooms
2 shallots, minced
2 tablespoons cognac
⅓ cup dry white wine
2 tablespoons chopped fresh
   tarragon

Serves 4	
Carb Level: Low	
Per serving:	
Carbohydrate:	8.1 g
Protein:	30.4 g

This recipe is forgiving of timing snafus. Keep the chicken covered in a warm oven; reheat the sauce and add the tarragon just before serving.

1. Preheat the oven to 350°.
2. Season the chicken with salt and pepper. Heat 1 teaspoon of the oil in a large nonstick sauté pan over medium heat. Lay the chicken breasts, skin side down, in the pan; cook for about 4 to 5 minutes, or until the skin is golden brown. Transfer the chicken, skin side up, to a nonstick baking pan. Reserve the sauté pan.
3. Bake the chicken, uncovered, for 20 minutes or until the juices run clear when the chicken is pierced with a knife.
4. While the chicken is baking, remove most of the fat from the sauté pan. Place over medium heat and add the carrot and onion. Cook until the vegetables begin to caramelize. Add the beef broth and raise the heat to high. Bring to a boil, reduce the heat, and simmer for 10 minutes, uncovered. Strain the broth though a fine-mesh sieve into a small bowl.
5. Warm the remaining 1 teaspoon of oil in the sauté pan over medium heat. Add the mushrooms and shallots and sauté until the mushrooms are golden. Season with salt and pepper. Remove the pan from the heat and add the cognac. Carefully ignite the cognac with a long match. Allow the flame to burn out, then add the wine. Return the pan to the heat.
6. Bring to a boil over medium heat. Allow to simmer for about 10 minutes, until the liquid is reduced by half. Add the reserved broth and simmer for 5 minutes or until the sauce is thick enough to coat the back of a spoon. Stir in the chopped tarragon.
7. Serve the sauce on top of the breasts.

Red Snapper
with Cayenne Tomato Sauce

Serves 1
Carb Level: Low

Per serving:

Carbohydrate:	2.2 g
Protein:	26.9 g

You can also heat the sauce for a nice touch.

∾

1 tablespoon olive oil
5 ounces red snapper fillet, skin on
2 tablespoons crème fraîche or sour cream
1 tablespoon minced chives
½ teaspoon sun-dried tomato paste
½ teaspoon cayenne pepper
1 teaspoon lemon juice
Salt and freshly ground black pepper to taste

1. Preheat oven to 375°.
2. Add the olive oil to a small ovenproof nonstick sauté pan over medium-high heat. Place the snapper fillet, skin side down, in the pan and cook until golden brown. Carefully turn the fillet over and place in the oven. Bake the snapper for about 6 minutes or until cooked through. To check for doneness, insert a thin-bladed knife in the thickest part of the fillet. The flesh should be flaky with no apparent translucence.
3. In a small bowl, mix together the crème fraîche, minced chives, tomato paste, cayenne, and lemon juice. Season with salt and pepper.
4. Serve the sauce over the snapper fillet.

What Is Clarified Butter?

Clarified butter is also known as drawn butter. Clarifying butter separates the milk solids and evaporates the water, leaving a clear golden liquid. Clarified butter has a higher heating point before smoking and also has a longer shelf life than regular butter. Clarified butter is used to sauté where a high heating point is needed.

Roasted Duck with Lemon

3 lemons
Salt
Freshly ground black pepper
4½-pound ready-to-cook duck
3 tablespoons butter

2 teaspoons sugar
2 tablespoons white wine
 vinegar
1 16-oz. can chicken stock
3 tablespoons dry sherry

Serves 6

Carb Level: Low

Per serving:

Carbohydrate:	5.1 g
Protein:	28.7 g

Meat left over from the duck carcass can be used in a crepe filling or as a duck salad on a bed of greens.

1. Preheat oven to 375°.
2. Cut the rind from 2 of the lemons as thinly as possible. Juice 1 of the lemons and set aside the juice. Separate the other lemon into segments and set aside. Cut the rind into narrow strips and cook in boiling water for 5 minutes. Rinse with cold water and pat dry.
3. Season the inside and outside of the duck with salt and pepper. Place half of the lemon rind and half of the butter in the cavity, then tie the legs together with a piece of white butcher's twine. Place the duck on a rack in a roasting pan just large enough to hold the duck without the skin touching the sides.
4. Roast the duck, uncovered, for about 1 hour and 15 minutes or until the leg meat begins to separate from the bone. (Cover the duck with a tent made of tin foil after about 45 minutes of cooking if the skin appears to be browning too rapidly.) Baste the duck with its natural juices during the roasting process. Let the duck rest for at least 30 minutes before carving.
5. In a medium-size saucepan over medium heat, cook the sugar and vinegar together, stirring often, until a caramel has formed. Add a little chicken stock and stir, scraping the bottom of the saucepan. Add the rest of the stock, the reserved lemon juice, and the remaining lemon rind strips. Add the dry sherry and any natural juices in the roasting pan from the duck; simmer over medium heat until the sauce is thick enough to coat the back of a spoon. Add the reserved lemon segments and the rest of the butter and simmer for another 5 minutes.
6. To serve, present slices of breast meat on a warmed plate with a drizzle of sauce over the top, or serve full quarters of the duck with the sauce presented on the side. Garnish with lemon slices.

Grilled Lamb Chops
with Provençal Roasted Tomatoes

Serves 4	
Carb Level: Low	

Per serving:

Carbohydrate:	8.9 g
Protein:	41.0 g

Use ripe, sun-warmed tomatoes for the best flavor. They also work well with grilled steaks or chicken.

ᔍ

For the lamb:

3 cloves garlic, minced (divided)
2 tablespoons olive oil
3 teaspoons fresh thyme leaves
4 sprigs fresh rosemary
Freshly ground black pepper
8 baby lamb chops
Salt

1. Place 2 of the minced garlic cloves in a mixing bowl. Add the olive oil, thyme, rosemary, and pepper; mix with a fork. Dredge lamb chops in the mixture and place the chops in a single layer in a shallow baking dish. Pour any remaining marinade over the chops. Cover and refrigerate for 4 hours.

Cooking with Wine
Wines are often reduced and used as a flavoring agent for many classical French sauces. One cup of white wine reduced by half contains 1.9 grams of carbohydrates.

(recipe continues on the next page)

Grilled Lamb Chops
with Provençal Roasted Tomatoes (continued)

For the tomatoes:

2 large ripe tomatoes, halved crosswise and seeded
2 teaspoons salt
2 tablespoons grated Parmesan cheese
2 tablespoons chopped fresh flat-leaf parsley
3 teaspoons fresh thyme leaves
3 tablespoons olive oil
2 cloves garlic, minced
Salt and freshly ground black pepper
4 sprigs fresh flatleaf parsley for garnish (optional)

1. Sprinkle the tomatoes with salt and put them, cut-side down, on a wire rack over a pan. Allow them to drain for about 15 minutes. In a small bowl combine the Parmesan, chopped parsley, thyme leaves, olive oil, garlic, and salt and pepper; stir to combine.
2. Preheat broiler on high.
3. Fit the tomatoes, cut-side up, into a small oiled baking dish just large enough to hold them. Sprinkle the tomatoes with the cheese and herb mixture. Broil for about 10 minutes or until the tomatoes have softened and the tops are golden brown. Cover with foil to keep warm.
4. Season both sides of the lamb chops with salt and pepper. Grill or broil for 3 minutes on each side for medium-rare (warm, pink center). Place 2 tomato halves in the center of each warm dinner plate and lay 2 chops over the tomatoes. Garnish with parsley sprigs.

Baked Haddock
with Parsley and Lemon

Serves 2
Carb Level: Low

Per serving:

Carbohydrate:	4.3 g
Protein:	49.3 g

Use the freshest fish you can get to make this recipe a sure hit.

∾

1 egg beaten with 1 tablespoon milk
³/₄–1 pound haddock fillet
2 tablespoons freshly grated Parmesan cheese
1 tablespoon bread crumbs
1 tablespoon olive oil
2 tablespoons butter, divided
2 tablespoons minced parsley
1 teaspoon grated lemon zest

1. Place the beaten egg mixture in a glass bowl and soak the fish in the egg wash for about 30 minutes, refrigerated.
2. Mix together the Parmesan and bread crumbs. Remove the fish from the egg wash, shaking off any excess, and dip it into the bread crumb mixture, lightly coating the fish.
3. Preheat the oven to 375°.
4. In a medium-size nonstick sauté pan with an ovenproof handle, heat the oil and 1 tablespoon of the butter together over medium heat until it just starts to foam. Add the fish and lightly brown the fillet on both sides. Place the sauté pan in the oven and bake for about 8 to 10 minutes or until the fish is cooked through. To check for doneness, insert a thin-bladed knife into the thickest part of the fish. The flesh should be flaky and there should be no trace of translucence.
5. Remove the fish from the sauté pan and keep it warm while preparing the sauce. Melt the remaining tablespoon of butter in the same sauté pan, scraping the bottom of the pan to loosen any browned bits from the fish. Add the parsley and lemon zest. Cook over medium heat, stirring constantly, until the butter is infused with the lemon flavor, about 1 to 2 minutes.
6. To serve, pour the butter sauce over each fillet and serve immediately.

Halibut with Porcinis, Shallots, and Tomatoes

¾ cup clam juice
1 cup water
1 bay leaf
10 black peppercorns
2 cloves garlic, crushed and peeled
½ ounce dried porcini mushrooms
⅓ cup olive oil
2 large shallots, minced

½ cup dry white wine
2–3 sprigs fresh tarragon or ¼ teaspoon dried tarragon
Salt and freshly ground black pepper taste
1 cup roughly chopped fresh or canned plum tomatoes (drained if canned)
4 (7–8 ounce) halibut steaks

Serves 4

Carb Level: Moderate

Per serving:

Carbohydrate:	19.6 g
Protein:	44.5 g

To make this recipe easier to prepare, premeasure and organize the ingredients before you begin.

∾

1. Combine the clam juice, water, bay leaf, peppercorns, and garlic in a medium-size saucepan. Bring to a boil and simmer gently, uncovered, over medium heat for about 10 minutes. Strain, discard solids, and set the stock aside.

2. Soak the dried porcini mushrooms in ½ cup of the prepared stock. Heat the olive oil in a large sauté pan over medium heat. Add the shallots and cook until tender. Drain and chop the porcinis (save and strain the mushroom soaking liquid) and add them to the shallots. Cook for about 1 minute. Add the wine, tarragon, mushroom soaking liquid, and the rest of the prepared stock. Bring to a boil and simmer until reduced by half.

3. Season the sauce with salt and pepper and add the tomatoes. Cook over medium heat for 2 to 3 minutes. Add the halibut fillets to the pan, cover, and simmer gently for about 5 minutes. Halibut is delicate, be careful not to over cook. To check for doneness, insert a thin-bladed knife into the thickest part of the fish. The flesh should be flaky and there should be no trace of translucence.

4. Use a large slotted spoon to move the fish to a warm platter. Adjust the seasoning of the sauce to taste. Add some fresh squeezed lemon juice if desired. After the fish is removed, the stock may be simmered, uncovered, over medium heat to concentrate the flavors. To serve, spoon the warm sauce over the fillets.

Lemon Chicken

Serves 4
Carb Level: Low

Per serving:

Carbohydrate:	7.8 g
Protein:	50.0 g

The lemon combined with the richness of skin-on roasted chicken is a true treat.

෴

1 (4 pound) roasting chicken
Salt and freshly ground black
*   pepper*
3 lemons

6 cloves garlic, peeled
½ medium onion, cut in half
Olive oil

1. Preheat oven to 375°.
2. Rinse the chicken and pat dry. Salt and pepper the inside cavity of the chicken. Pierce the lemons all over with a fork and place them in the cavity along with the garlic and onion pieces. Truss the chicken by tying the legs together with a piece of butcher's twine and tucking in the wing tips to keep them from overcooking. Rub the chicken with olive oil and season with salt and freshly ground black pepper. Place the chicken on a rack in a baking dish just large enough to hold the chicken without it touching the sides.
3. Bake for about 1 to 1½ hours, until the leg meat pulls easily from the bone. Check the chicken occasionally during the cooking process and baste it with the natural juices from the pan. (Make a tent out of tin foil and place it over the chicken if the skin seems to be browning too rapidly.)
4. When the chicken is ready, discard the stuffing and let the chicken rest, tented with tin foil, for about 10 to 15 minutes. Carve and serve with the natural pan juices.

A Twist on the Sauce

Whisk a touch of heavy cream with a pinch of cayenne pepper in with the natural pan juices to enrich the sauce. Don't forget to pick up all the caramelized brown bits at the bottom of the roasting pan for the best flavor. Heat the sauce and simmer for a few minutes to slightly thicken and to allow the flavors to meld.

Beef Provençal

¼ pound bacon, chopped

2 pounds boneless chuck or rump roast, cut into 2-inch cubes

Salt and freshly ground black pepper to taste

2 medium onions, peeled and quartered

1 small fennel bulb, trimmed and thinly sliced

1 head garlic, separated into cloves and peeled

6 large strips of orange zest, pith removed

1 bay leaf

Pinch of dried basil

Pinch of dried thyme

Pinch of dried parsley

1 cup red wine (merlot or cabernet)

1 cup beef broth

12 whole black olives, pitted (Mediterranean style preferably)

Serves 4	
Carb Level: Moderate	
Per serving:	
Carbohydrate:	13.7 g
Protein:	48.7 g

Great for advance preparation—the flavors improve if allowed to sit refrigerated overnight. Or freeze portions to save even longer.

1. Using a large sauté pan with a lid, cook the bacon over medium heat until crispy. Remove the bacon with a slotted spoon and set aside. Remove ½ of the bacon fat and reserve. Season the beef with salt and pepper.

2. Heat the pan over medium-high and cook the onions until lightly browned. Add the meat and brown on all sides. Add additional bacon fat as needed. Remove the meat and onions and any accumulated juices and set aside.

3. Reheat the sauté pan over medium-high heat with a little more of the bacon fat. Add the fennel, garlic cloves, orange zest, bay leaf, and dried herbs. Cook until the vegetables are tender. Add the meat and onions, red wine, and the beef broth. Bring the stew to a simmer and cook, covered, over very low heat. Braise for about 2 hours or until the meat begins to fall apart. Skim off any fat that rises to the top.

4. Serve the stew in warm bowls garnished with the olives and the crispy bacon.

Trout Grenobloise

Serves 4

Carb Level: Moderate

Per serving:

Carbohydrate:	14.9 g
Protein:	18.2 g

Keep the cream from curdling by using it at room temperature, keeping the pan off the heat, and adding the cream slowly.

1 lemon
4 (4-ounce) trout fillets, boned, skin-on
Salt and freshly ground black pepper to taste
1 teaspoon canola oil
1 teaspoon, plus 1 tablespoon unsalted butter
2 tablespoons capers, well drained

2 tablespoons chopped fresh flat-leaf parsley
3 tablespoons heavy cream, room temperature
4 slices lemon for garnish
4 sprigs fresh flat-leaf parsley for garnish

1. Peel the lemon, removing all of the white pith. Cut the flesh into a small dice, discarding any seeds.
2. Season the trout fillets with salt and pepper and keep refrigerated until ready to use.
3. Combine the oil and 1 teaspoon of the butter in a large nonstick sauté pan over medium-high heat. When the pan is hot, place the fillets, skin side down, in the pan. Cook for about 1 to 1½ minutes, until golden brown. Carefully turn the fillets over with a long spatula and cook for another 2 minutes or until cooked through.
4. Transfer the fillets to warm plates and keep in warm spot.
5. Using the same sauté pan, wipe out the interior of the pan with a paper towel. Return the pan to medium heat and add the remaining tablespoon of butter. Cook until the butter just begins to brown. Remove the pan from the heat and stir in the capers, parsley, and diced lemon. Very slowly, add the cream, a few drops at a time, and whisk to incorporate. Return the pan to the heat just to warm the sauce through.
6. Spoon the mixture over the trout fillets and garnish with a slice of lemon and a sprig of parsley.

Veal Stew Blanquette

1½ pounds veal stew meat, trimmed of all fat and cut into 1-inch cubes
Salt
1 small onion, quartered with root intact
1 rib celery, cut in half lengthwise
½ leek, white part only, washed well and cut in half lengthwise
1 clove garlic, crushed
2 sprigs fresh thyme
2 sprigs fresh flat-leaf parsley
1 bay leaf
¼ teaspoon paprika
Freshly ground black pepper
½ teaspoon unsalted butter
1 tablespoon cornstarch
1½ cups milk
¼ cup sour cream
2 tablespoons chopped fresh flat-leaf parsley for garnish

Serves 4

Carb Level: Moderate

Per serving:

Carbohydrate:	12.3 g
Protein:	39.5 g

This French classic usually includes onions, eliminated here to keep the carb count within reason.

~

1. Blanch the veal: Rinse the veal cubes under cold running water. Place the meat in a large saucepan and add cold water to cover by about 1 inch. Bring to a boil over high heat. Remove the pan from the heat and drain well. Rinse the veal under cold running water. Rinse out the saucepan.
2. Return the veal to the saucepan and add cold water to cover by about 1 inch. Season with salt. Bring just to a simmer over medium-high heat. Do not allow the mixture to boil. Carefully skim off and discard any fat that rises to the top.
3. Add the onion, celery, leek, garlic, thyme, parsley sprigs, bay leaf, paprika, and pepper. Bring to a simmer over medium-high heat. Reduce the heat to medium-low and allow the stew to simmer for 45 to 60 minutes or until the veal is very tender.
4. Strain the veal mixture though a colander, reserving the cooking liquid. Transfer the veal to a plate.
5. Strain the liquid through a fine-mesh sieve into a large saucepan. Add butter and bring to a simmer over medium heat.
6. Place the cornstarch in a small bowl. Gradually whisk in the milk until smooth. Whisk into the cooking liquid and bring to a boil. When the liquid has thickened, add the reserved veal. Cook until heated through. Gently stir in the sour cream.
7. Ladle stew into warm shallow bowls and garnish with the chopped parsley.

CHAPTER 4

Italian Food

Portobellos Stuffed with Basil and Salmon on Arugula Leaves ❖ — 54

Veal Cutlets with Ricotta Cheese and Spinach — 55

Broiled Scallops with Apple-Wood Smoked Bacon — 56

Veal Osso Buco — 57

Venetian Liver and Onions ❖ — 58

Rabbit and Herb Stew — 59

Chicken Cacciatore — 60

Baked Ocean Perch with Black Olives and Capers — 61

Chicken Breast Paillards Layered with Prosciutto and Cheese ❖ — 62

Tuscan Lamb Chops ❖ — 63

Veal Scallops with Marsala Wine — 64

Broiled Marinated Steak-Bistecca ❖ — 65

Pork Chops Braised in White Wine — 66

Tomato Sauce ❖ — 67

❖ **Indicates Easy Recipe** ❖

Portobellos Stuffed
with Basil and Salmon on Arugula Leaves

Serves 2
Carb Level: Low

Per serving:	
Carbohydrate:	7.3 g
Protein:	28.2 g

Baby organic arugula leaves have a mild peppery bite and wonderful texture that complement this dish.

ও

2 large portobello mushroom
    caps
3 teaspoons sunflower oil or
    light olive oil
Salt and freshly ground black
    pepper to taste
2 tablespoons minced scallion
2 cloves garlic, minced
¼ cup fresh basil leaves,
    julienned

3 tablespoons cream cheese
½ pound salmon, skinned,
    boned, and chopped into
    medium cubes
10 ounces fresh arugula leaves,
    stemmed

1. Preheat oven to 375°.
2. Brush the mushrooms with the oil and season with salt and pepper. Place the mushrooms on a foil-covered baking sheet, lightly oiled, stem side up. Roast for about 20 to 30 minutes, until tender when pierced with a fork, but not shriveled.
3. Mix together the scallion, garlic, basil, and cream cheese in a small bowl. Split the salmon into 2 equal portions and place each piece on a mushroom cap. Top with the cream cheese mixture. Season with salt and freshly ground black pepper.
4. Bake the stuffed mushroom, uncovered, for about 20 to 25 minutes, until the cream cheese is bubbly and starting to brown on top and the salmon is cooked through. Serve each mushroom cap on a bed of arugula leaves.

Green Facts

Arugula is also known as rocket or rugula. The tender baby leaves are best, featuring a peppery bite. The larger leaves are somewhat bitter. Fresh arugula contains a fair amount of grit, so the leaves should be rinsed several times before using. Arugula is a good source of iron as well as vitamins A and C.

Veal Cutlets
with Ricotta Cheese and Spinach

*¾ pound veal scaloppini
(pounded veal cutlets)
2 eggs beaten with a pinch of
salt and pepper
2 tablespoons butter
10 ounces frozen chopped
spinach, thawed, drained,
and moisture squeezed out
2 cloves garlic, minced*

*½ cup ricotta cheese
3 tablespoons sour cream
Pinch of freshly grated nutmeg
Salt and freshly ground black
pepper to taste
1 tablespoon freshly grated
Parmesan cheese, plus extra
for garnish*

Serves 2
Carb Level: Low

Per serving:	
Carbohydrate:	9.5 g
Protein:	46.0 g

Ricotta is a rich fresh cheese, with 3.8 carbohydrates per ½ cup. It is slightly grainy but smoother and a touch sweeter than cottage cheese.

1. Soak the veal in the beaten egg for 30 minutes.
2. Melt the butter in a large sauté pan over medium-high heat; sauté the spinach and garlic, uncovered, for about 3 to 5 minutes. Season with salt and pepper. Remove the spinach from skillet and set aside.
3. Preheat the oven to 375°.
4. In a large nonstick skillet, over low heat, add half of the veal slices 1 at a time and cook just long enough to set the egg coating on both sides. Remove the slices as they are done and place in a 2-quart ovenproof casserole dish.
5. Put the ricotta and sour cream in a food processor (or a blender) with a pinch of nutmeg, salt and pepper, and the grated Parmesan; blend until smooth. Spread half of the cheese mixture over the veal with the back of a spoon. Layer ½ cup of the spinach on top.
6. Cook the rest of the scaloppini and layer it on top of the spinach in the casserole dish. Layer the other ½ cup spinach and spread the rest of the cheese on top. Bake for about 30 minutes or until the cheese topping is set. Cut and serve like a lasagna, or scoop with a large spoon. Sprinkle a little Parmesan cheese on top to garnish.

Broiled Scallops
with Apple-Wood Smoked Bacon

Serves 4

Carb Level: Low

Per serving:

Carbohydrate:	3.4 g
Protein:	19.4 g

This is a delicious appetizer or first course dish. If serving as an appetizer, use skewers instead of toothpicks.

6 slices of apple-wood smoked bacon, cut in half
12 large scallops, patted dry
1 tablespoon finely grated lemon zest
1 sprig fresh rosemary, finely minced
1/3 cup pitted and chopped black olives
2 plum tomatoes, peeled, seeded, and diced
2 tablespoons drained capers
1 clove garlic, chopped
2 tablespoons chopped fresh chives, divided
Extra-virgin olive oil

1. Preheat oven to 350°.
2. Place the bacon on a nonstick baking sheet and precook for about 8 minutes. The bacon should be almost fully cooked but still pliable. Drain the bacon on paper towels; discard the fat from the baking sheet. Lay the bacon slices on a clean flat work surface. Sprinkle the scallops with the lemon zest and rosemary and place 1 on each piece of bacon. Wrap the bacon around the scallop and secure with a toothpick.
3. Mix the next 4 ingredients and 1 tablespoon of the chives in a small bowl. Pour in enough olive oil to glaze the mixture together, mix to combine.
4. Brush the wrapped scallops with the olive oil and brown under a hot broiler or fry in a hot nonstick skillet for 1 to 2 minutes on each side, until slightly caramelized. Remove the toothpick, and serve the scallops with a dollop of the olive relish. Sprinkle with the remaining chives.

Antipasto Platters

Antipasto literally means "before the pasta." These platters are traditionally served before a hearty pasta course, but can also be a main course all on their own. The platters should include cheeses; marinated, roasted, or grilled vegetables; smoked meats; and olives. The platter may also include fish or shellfish.

Veal Osso Buco

4 veal shank cross cuts, about
   1½ inches thick (osso buco)
Salt and freshly ground black
   pepper to taste
Oil for cooking
3 tablespoons unsalted butter
1 carrot, sliced
1 stalk celery, sliced
1 onion, sliced
4 cloves garlic, chopped
8 tomatoes, peeled, seeded,
   and chopped

1 cup dry white wine
2 bay leaves
3 sprigs fresh thyme
1 quart beef stock or water
2 tablespoons chopped fresh
   parsley
1 teaspoon finely grated
   orange zest
1 teaspoon finely grated lemon
   zest

Serves 4
Carb Level: Moderate

Per serving:

Carbohydrate:	19.6 g
Protein:	51.1 g

Time is the key ingredient in making this classic, which is a staple menu item in many Italian restaurants.

1. Preheat oven to 350°.
2. Trim the meat of any excess fat. Season with salt and pepper. Using a Dutch oven, heat a little oil over high heat and brown the veal on both sides, in batches if necessary. Remove the shanks from the Dutch oven and set aside.
3. Reduce the heat to medium-high and melt the butter in the same pot; cook the carrot, celery, and onion for 3 minutes. Add the garlic and mix well. Add the chopped tomatoes and cook for 5 minutes. Add the white wine, bay leaves, and thyme sprigs; cook for another 5 minutes. Add the stock and the browned meat; bring to a simmer, season with salt and pepper, and cover. Transfer to the oven and bake for 1½ hours or until the meat is tender (the shank should begin to fall apart somewhat).
4. Use a slotted spoon to transfer the meat to a serving platter, cover, and keep warm. Return the Dutch oven to the stovetop. Heat the cooking liquid and vegetables and bring to a boil. Skim off any fat or foam that rises to the top. Cook for 20 to 25 minutes or until the sauce has thickened and coats the back of the spoon. Stir in the parsley, orange and lemon zest, and season to taste. Simmer for another 5 minutes, then pour over the meat and serve immediately.

Venetian Liver and Onions

Serves 4
Carb Level: Moderate
Per serving:
Carbohydrate: 11.6 g
Protein: 21.2 g

Liver is a great source of protein, vitamin A, and iron.

&

1 pound calf's liver, sliced into medallions
Vegetable oil for cooking
2 medium-size yellow onions, thinly sliced

Salt and freshly ground black pepper to taste

1. Make sure the liver is completely free of veins and remove any of the membrane that may still be attached. (Usually your butcher will do all of this for you.)
2. Heat 2 to 3 tablespoons of oil in a large nonstick skillet on high heat and add the onion and a large pinch of salt. Reduce to medium heat and cook for 20 to 30 minutes or until the onions are completely soft and golden brown. Remove the onions from the pan and set aside.
3. Add a little more oil to the skillet if necessary and heat until almost smoking. Fry the liver in small batches, just enough to cover the base of the pan, for about 1 to 2 minutes or until it has changed color from pink to brown. (*Hint:* Make sure your pan is very hot, as the liver must fry quickly to ensure that it does not stick or overcook.) Turn the medallions and cook for about 1 minute. Transfer each batch to a warm plate and season to taste with salt and pepper.
4. Return all the liver to the pan, add the cooked onions, and toss to combine, but do not cook further. Transfer to a warm serving plate and serve immediately.

Rabbit and Herb Stew

1 (2½-pound) rabbit, cut into
   8 pieces
1 cup all-purpose flour, seasoned with salt and pepper
1 cup canola oil
1 onion, finely chopped
⅔ cup sliced button mush-
   rooms
1 teaspoon tomato paste

1 clove garlic, chopped
Salt and freshly ground black
   pepper to taste
2 cups chicken stock
8 ripe tomatoes, peeled,
   seeded, and chopped
¼ cup chopped fresh herbs
   (rosemary, marjoram,
   parsley, etc.)

Serves 4
Carb Level: Moderate

Per serving:	
Carbohydrate:	16.7 g
Protein:	14.1 g

Many supermarkets carry rabbit in the freezer section. You can prepare this stew ahead and allow the flavors to meld overnight.

1. Coat the rabbit in the flour, shaking off any excess. Heat about ½ cup of the oil in a large skillet on high heat. Brown the rabbit on all sides. Remove from the pan with a slotted spoon and drain on paper towels. (Cook the rabbit in batches if necessary to avoid crowding the pan.)
2. Add the onion to the pan and cook over low heat until soft. Increase heat and add the mushrooms. Continue to cook, stirring frequently, for about 5 minutes. Add the tomato paste and garlic, and stir to mix. Transfer to flameproof casserole dish or a Dutch oven, add the rabbit, and season with the salt and pepper.
3. Add the stock (it should be enough to barely cover the rabbit) and simmer gently on the stovetop for 45 minutes.
4. Add the tomatoes and cook for another 10 minutes. Add the chopped fresh herbs and season to taste. (The meat should be tender and should be separating from the bone.) Serve the meat on a platter or on individual dishes with the sauce spooned over.

Fresh Herbs or Dried Ones?

Fresh herbs have flavors that are delicate and intense. They should be added to a dish at the end of the cooking process to preserve their flavor. Dried herbs have a stronger, more concentrated flavor, so you'll want to add them early in the preparation of a dish. Crush them up before adding them to extract more of their flavor.

Chicken Cacciatore

Serves 4
Carb Level: Moderate

Per serving:	
Carbohydrate:	17.4 g
Protein:	46.1 g

The vegetables increase the carb count on this recipe to a moderate level.

∾

¼ cup olive oil
1 (3½-pound) chicken, cut into 8 pieces
Salt and freshly ground black pepper
2 medium onions, thinly sliced into rings
3 cloves garlic, finely chopped
1¼ cups thinly sliced button mushrooms
1 small green bell pepper, thinly sliced
¼ cup tomato paste
¾ cup dry white wine
16 ounces canned plum tomatoes
½ teaspoon dried rosemary
½ teaspoon dried oregano
Freshly grated Parmesan cheese for garnish

1. Heat the olive oil in a large skillet on high heat to almost smoking. Season the chicken with salt and pepper, and fry it, skin-side down, for 5 minutes or until lightly browned. Turn over and brown the other side. Remove the chicken pieces with a slotted spoon and set aside.

2. Reduce heat to medium. Add the onions to the pan and cook for 5 minutes, then add the garlic, mushrooms, and green pepper. Cook for another 3 to 4 minutes or until the onions are golden, stirring frequently. Mix in the tomato paste and white wine and cook for 1 to 2 minutes, then add the tomatoes, breaking them down with a wooden spoon. Sprinkle in the rosemary and oregano and return the chicken to the pan. Season with salt and pepper, cover, and simmer for 30 minutes, stirring occasionally.

3. Check the chicken to ensure it is cooked and tender. If it is still resistant when pierced with a fork, cover and cook for another 10 minutes. The leg meat should easily pull away from the bone. Using a slotted spoon, transfer the chicken pieces to a serving plate; keep warm. If the sauce appears too liquid, allow it to lightly boil, uncovered, for 5 minutes to slightly thicken. Season to taste, then pour over the chicken. Serve immediately. Garnish with freshly grated Parmesan cheese.

Baked Ocean Perch
with Black Olives and Capers

$^{1}/_{4}$ cup olive oil

6 tablespoons butter, divided

2 teaspoons dried oregano

Freshly ground black pepper

2 pounds ocean perch,
    cleaned, skin on

3 tablespoons capers, thor-
    oughly washed and drained

2 tablespoons slivered black
    olives

Salt

2 tablespoons lemon juice

2 tablespoons finely chopped
    fresh flat-leaf parsley

Serves 4	
Carb Level: Low	
Per serving:	
Carbohydrate:	2.1 g
Protein:	16.3 g

Delicate ocean perch is perfectly paired in this great trio of Mediterranean flavors.

1. In a large nonstick skillet heat the oil and 2 tablespoons of the butter over medium heat until it begins to sizzle. Stir in the oregano and a few grindings of black pepper. Add the fish, skin side down. Cook for about 3 to 4 minutes on each side. With a slotted spatula, carefully transfer the fish to a heated platter.

2. Reduce heat to low and add the remaining 4 tablespoons of butter to the skillet; heat until it turns a light amber brown, but be careful not to burn it. Stir in the capers and olives. Remove the skillet from the heat and stir in the lemon juice and parsley. Gently heat and stir to mix; pour over the fish and serve immediately

The Flavor of a Caper

Capers have an intense salty flavor that lends a burst of flavor in many sauces and condiments. They are usually stored and sold in a brine and should be rinsed in cold running water before using.

Chicken Breast Paillards Layered with Prosciutto and Cheese

Serves 4
Carb Level: Low

Per serving:

Carbohydrate:	7.2 g
Protein:	112.6 g

You can use any leftovers from this dish the next day sliced on top of a salad for a antipasto-style treat.

∾

4 (⅓- to ½-pound) skinless, boneless chicken breasts
Salt and freshly ground black pepper to taste
3 tablespoons all-purpose flour
3 tablespoons butter
2 tablespoons oil

8 thin (2-inch-wide, 4-inch-long) slices prosciutto
8 thin (2-inch-wide, 4-inch-long) slices imported fontina or Bel Paese cheese
4 teaspoons freshly grated imported Parmesan cheese
¼ cup chicken stock

1. Preheat oven to 350°.
2. With a very sharp knife, carefully slice each chicken breast horizontally to make 8 thin slices. Lay them an inch or so apart in between 2 sheets of wax paper. Pound the chicken slices lightly with the flat side of a cleaver or the bottom of a heavy bottle to flatten them somewhat. Strip off the paper.
3. Season the slices with salt and a few grindings of black pepper, then dip them in flour and shake off the excess. In a heavy, large nonstick skillet, melt the butter with the oil over moderate heat. Brown the chicken (both sides) to a light golden color, 3 or 4 slices at a time. Do not overcook them.
4. Transfer the chicken paillards to a shallow buttered baking dish large enough to hold them without overcrowding. Place a slice of prosciutto and then a slice of cheese on each. Sprinkle them with the Parmesan and drizzle the chicken stock over the top. Bake uncovered in the middle of the oven for 10 minutes or until the cheese is melted and lightly browned. Serve immediately.

Tuscan Lamb Chops

*4 (1-inch-thick) lamb rib chops
(1½ pounds total)*
2 teaspoons olive oil
3 cloves garlic, minced
*1 (8-ounce) can Italian-style
stewed tomatoes, undrained*

1 tablespoon balsamic vinegar
*2 teaspoons finely chopped
fresh rosemary*

Serves 2
Carb Level: Moderate

Per serving:	
Carbohydrate:	12.8 g
Protein:	64.9 g

Classic flavors blend
well in this easy,
1-skillet dinner entrée.

❦

1. Trim any excess fat from the chops. Heat the oil in a large nonstick sauté pan over medium-high heat. Cook the chops for about 6 minutes on each side for medium doneness, turning once. Transfer the chops to a plate; keep warm.
2. Stir the garlic into the drippings in the skillet; cook, stirring constantly, for 1 minute. Add the tomatoes, vinegar, and rosemary. Bring to a boil; reduce heat and simmer, uncovered, for 3 minutes or until it is fairly thick consistency. Spoon sauce over the chops and serve immediately.

Veal Scallops with Marsala Wine

Serves 4
Carb Level: Low

Per serving:	
Carbohydrate:	5.2 g
Protein:	23.7 g

Marsala wine is fortified with brandy and is commonly used in cooking.

❧

1½ pounds veal scallops, sliced ³/₈-inch thick
Salt and freshly ground black pepper to taste
3 tablespoons all-purpose flour
2 tablespoons butter

3 tablespoons olive oil
½ cup dry Marsala wine
½ cup chicken or beef stock, divided
2 tablespoons butter, softened

1. Pound the veal scallops to ¼-inch thick. Season with salt and pepper, then dip them in flour and vigorously shake off the excess. In a large nonstick skillet, melt 2 tablespoons of butter with the olive oil over medium heat. When the foam subsides, add the scallops, 3 or 4 at a time, and brown them for about 3 minutes on each side. As they are done, transfer them to a plate; keep warm.

2. Pour off most of the fat from the skillet, leaving a thin film on the bottom (keeping all the browned meat scraps). Add the Marsala and ¼ cup of stock and boil the liquid briskly over high heat for 1 to 2 minutes to deglaze the pan. Return the veal to the skillet, cover the pan, and simmer over low heat for 10 to 15 minutes.

3. Transfer the veal scallops to a heated platter. Add the remaining ¼ cup of stock to the skillet with the wine-stock mixture and boil briskly, scraping in the browned bits sticking to the sides of the pan. When the sauce has reduced considerably and has the consistency of a syrupy glaze, adjust salt and pepper to taste. Remove the pan from the heat, stir in the soft butter, and pour the sauce over the scallops. Serve immediately.

Storing Butter

Butter rapidly absorbs flavors. Regular butter can be stored in the refrigerator for up to one month, wrapped airtight. Unsalted butter should be stored for no longer than two weeks in the refrigerator.

Broiled Marinated Steak-Bistecca

¾ cup olive oil
¼ cup red wine vinegar
2 tablespoons finely chopped
  fresh flat-leaf parsley
½ teaspoon finely chopped
  garlic
½ teaspoon dried oregano

2½–3 pound (1-inch-thick)
  T-bone, porterhouse,
  or sirloin steak
Salt and freshly ground black
  pepper to taste

Serves 4
Carb Level: Low

Per serving:

Carbohydrate:	1.2 g
Protein:	48.8 g

These steaks also work great on the grill.

1. In a shallow baking dish large enough to hold the steak comfortably, combine the olive oil, vinegar, parsley, garlic, and oregano. Lay the steak in the marinade and turn it to coat both sides completely. Let the steak marinate for at least 6 hours in the refrigerator, turning it every so often.
2. Preheat the broiler.
3. Remove the steak from the baking dish (discard the marinade). Broil it 3 inches from the heat for about 4 minutes on each side or until it is done to your taste. Remove from broiler and sprinkle with salt and pepper. Let the steak rest for 5 minutes before carving. Slice into ½-inch strips, cutting slightly on the bias. Transfer the steak to a warmed platter and serve immediately.

The Low-Down on Olive Oil

The best-quality olive oil is cold-pressed extra-virgin. Cold pressing is a natural, chemical-free process that involves only pressure and no additives. The result is an olive oil with low acidity.

Pork Chops Braised in White Wine

Serves 4
Carb Level: Low

Per serving:

Carbohydrate:	1.4 g
Protein:	29.9 g

Great served with Creamed Spinach (see recipe on page 138).

෨

1 tablespoon chopped fresh sage leaves

1 tablespoon chopped fresh rosemary leaves

1 tablespoon chopped fresh basil leaves

1 teaspoon finely chopped garlic

1 teaspoon salt

Freshly ground black pepper

4 tablespoons olive oil, divided

4 (1-inch-thick) center-cut loin pork chops

2 tablespoons butter

¾ cup dry white wine, divided

1 tablespoon finely chopped fresh Italian flat-leaf parsley

1. In a medium-size mixing bowl, combine the sage, rosemary, basil, garlic, salt, and a few grindings of pepper with 2 tablespoons of the olive oil. Dredge the chops in the herb mixture, ensuring both sides are evenly coated. In a large heavy-bottomed skillet, melt the butter with the remaining 2 tablespoons of olive oil over medium heat. When the foam subsides, add the chops and brown them for 2 to 3 minutes on each side, turning them carefully with tongs. When the chops are golden brown, remove them from the pan to a platter; keep warm.

2. Pour off all but a thin film of fat from the bottom of the skillet, retaining the browned bits on the bottom of the pan. Add ½ cup of the white wine and bring to a boil to deglaze the pan. Return the chops to the pan, cover, and reduce the heat to the barest simmer. Cook the chops for 25 to 30 minutes, or until they are tender when pierced with the tip of a sharp knife.

3. Transfer the chops to a heated serving platter. Add the remaining ¼ cup of wine to the skillet. Boil it briskly over high heat, stirring and scraping in any brown bits that cling to the bottom and sides of the pan, until it has reduced to a few tablespoons of syrupy glaze. Remove the skillet from the heat. Adjust seasoning to taste and stir in the parsley. Pour the sauce over the pork chops and serve.

Tomato Sauce

1 medium onion chopped
3 cloves garlic, finely chopped
3 tablespoons extra-virgin
   olive oil
1 (28-ounce) can crushed
   tomatoes in purée
1 (15-ounce) can tomato sauce
   with no added sugar

1 teaspoon baking soda
2/3 cup fresh chopped herbs,
   including basil, thyme, and
   parsley
Salt and freshly ground black
   pepper to taste

Makes 5 cups

Carb Level: Low

Per serving:

Carbohydrate:	8.1 g
Protein:	1.5 g

A great simple sauce that freezes well. It makes a nice topping for red meats or chicken.

1. In a medium-size skillet sauté the onion and garlic in the olive oil over medium heat until tender. Add the crushed tomatoes and tomato sauce, stirring to mix. Continue to stir to prevent scorching.
2. Add the baking soda and fresh herbs, continuing to stir. Lower heat to a simmer and add salt and pepper to taste. Simmer for 15 minutes, stirring frequently.

 The Carb Counts of Tomatoes

Tomato juice (6 ounces)	8 g
Red, ripe raw tomatoes (1 cup)	8 g
Canned, stewed tomatoes (1 cup)	16 g
Canned tomato sauce (1/2 cup)	9 g
Canned tomato paste (1/4 cup)	12.5 g

CHAPTER 5

Mexican Specialties

Chickens Stuffed with Chorizo and Spinach	70
Spicy Pork Roast ❖	71
Halibut Ceviche with Herbs ❖	72
Classic Gazpacho ❖	73
Fiesta Salsa ❖	74
Garlic Shrimp with Salsa ❖	74
Drunken Chicken ❖	75
Pompano with Salsa Fresca ❖	76
Guacamole ❖	77
Mexican Tomato Salad ❖	78

❖ **Indicates Easy Recipe** ❖

Chickens Stuffed with Chorizo and Spinach

Serves 4

Carb Level: Moderate

Per serving:

Carbohydrate:	11.6 g
Protein:	90.1 g

You can find annatto, or achiote, paste in Mexican specialty stores.

2 (3-pound) chickens
1 package annatto (also called "achiote") paste
½ cup olive oil
1 teaspoon toasted cumin
1 teaspoon ground coriander
1 teaspoon Mexican oregano
5 tablespoons chopped garlic, divided
4 large links of hard dried Spanish chorizo

1 Spanish onion, diced
1 12–14 oz. box frozen chopped spinach, thawed and drained
½ cup chicken stock
2 tablespoons sliced green olives, drained
Salt and freshly ground black pepper

1. Rinse the chickens under cold running water and pat dry with paper towels, including the cavities. In a food processor, combine the annatto paste, olive oil, cumin, coriander, oregano, and 1 tablespoon of the garlic; purée to a paste. Wearing plastic gloves (the achiote will stain your fingers), rub the paste inside the chicken, under the skin, and on the outside. Marinate in the refrigerator overnight.

2. Preheat oven to 375°.

3. In a large sauté pan, over medium-high heat, cook the chorizo and onion for about 5 to 8 minutes, until it starts to brown. Add the remaining 4 tablespoons of garlic; cook for 2 minutes. Add the spinach and the chicken stock and cook for another 4 to 5 minutes. Add the green olives and salt and pepper. Allow the filling to cool before stuffing the chickens.

4. Divide the stuffing equally between the cavities of the 2 chickens. Place them in a roasting pan on top of a wire rack. Roast for about 1 to 1½ hours or until the leg meat starts to pull away from the bone. The internal temperature should reach between 160 to 165°. Allow the chicken to rest in a warm place under a tin foil tent for about 20 minutes until ready to serve.

Spicy Pork Roast

¼ cup olive oil
¼ cup chili powder
¼ cup chili flakes
2 tablespoons oregano
1 tablespoon seasoned salt
1 tablespoon ground cumin
2 tablespoons fresh garlic, crushed
¼ cup chopped cilantro leaves
¼ cup chopped parsley leaves
2 tablespoons black pepper

1 cup chopped scallions
1 cup chopped Spanish onions
2 cups chicken or vegetable broth
6–8 pounds pork loin, cut into 2- to 3-inch cubes

Serves 12
Carb Level: Low

Per serving:	
Carbohydrate:	8.3 g
Protein:	55.2 g

Make a large batch and freeze some for later. It makes a great, filling winter meal.

∾

1. In a large bowl, mix together all the ingredients *except* the broth and pork. Add the pork, mix to ensure the meat is evenly coated, and allow to marinate in the refrigerator for about 4 hours.
2. Preheat the oven to 350°.
3. Place all the ingredients in a Dutch oven and add the broth. Roast, covered, for about 3½ to 4 hours or until the pork is very tender. Adjust seasoning to taste. Be careful not to stir too much, as the meat will start to come apart. Serve family style.

Do Onions Make You Cry?

Refrigerating an onion before chopping it will help keep your eyes from watering.

Halibut Ceviche with Herbs

Makes 8 appetizer portions
Carb Level: Low

Per serving:

Carbohydrate:	9.0 g
Protein:	12.7 g

The acid from the lime juice actually cooks the fish.

❧

1 pound very fresh halibut
½ cup freshly squeezed lime juice
1½ cups spicy tomato juice
1 ripe mango, peeled, seeded, and medium diced
8 teaspoons (or to taste) hot pepper sauce
1 tablespoon honey
8 teaspoons very finely minced green chili

¾ cup finely chopped herbs (mint, parsley, chervil, chives, cilantro, etc.), plus extra herb leaves for garnish
Salt and freshly ground black pepper to taste
Extra-virgin olive oil for drizzling

1. Using a sharp knife, cut the halibut into thin slices. In a bowl, mix the fish with the lime juice and allow to sit for 10 minutes at room temperature.
2. Remove the fish from the lime juice; discard the juice. Add all the remaining ingredients except the olive oil; mix to combine. Keep refrigerated until read to serve.
3. When ready to serve, drizzle a little oil around the ceviche and garnish with fresh herb leaves.

Citrus Juice and Carbohydrates

Note the carbohydrate counts for ¼ cup of the following freshly squeezed citrus juices:

Freshly squeezed lemon juice	5.3 g
Freshly squeezed lime juice	5.5 g
Freshly squeezed orange juice	6.5 g

Classic Gazpacho

1½ pounds red bell peppers
1 pound ripe tomatoes
1 pound cucumbers
2 medium cloves garlic, peeled
1 cup chopped sweet onion
¼ cup extra-virgin olive oil
¼ cup sherry vinegar

2 tablespoons good-quality
  tomato paste
Salt and freshly ground black
  pepper to taste
Fresh cilantro leaves and
  lemon wedges for garnish

Serves 6
Carb Level: Moderate
Per serving:

Carbohydrate:	16.4 g
Protein:	2.9 g

A refreshing summer treat when served in a chilled glass mug or bowl.

1. Roast the peppers over an open flame or under the broiler, turning often, until the skins are completely charred. Transfer the peppers to a bowl and cover with plastic wrap. Allow them to sit for about 15 minutes or until they are cool enough to handle. Rub off all of the charred skin carefully. Save any juices that may have accumulated in the bowl. (You can rinse the peppers under running water if desired, but you will loose some of the oils, which enhance the flavor.) Cut around the stem and pull it out. Scoop out the seeds with a spoon and add the peppers to the work bowl of a food processor.
2. Cut out and discard the stems of the tomatoes. Place the tomatoes in a pot of boiling water for only 30 seconds. Use a slotted spoon to remove the tomatoes from the boiling water and plunge them in a bowl of ice water. (This will stop the cooking process.) Skin and seed the tomatoes. Cut them into quarters and add to the work bowl. Discard the skin and seeds but save any residual juice.
3. Peel the cucumbers and cut them in half lengthwise. Scoop out the seeds (a teaspoon is a good tool for this task). Cut the cucumbers into chunks and add them to the food processor work bowl. Add the garlic, onion, olive oil, vinegar, and tomato paste to the food processor. Add the reserved tomato and pepper juices. Process for at least 2 minutes or until smooth. Season with salt and pepper to taste.
4. Place the gazpacho in a bowl, covered, and refrigerate for 2 to 4 hours. Classic gazpacho calls for straining the soup through a fine-mesh strainer. Serve in cold bowls and garnish with fresh cilantro leaves and wedges of fresh lemon.

Makes 2 cups
Carb Level: Moderate
Per serving:
Carbohydrate: 15.5 g
Protein: 1.7 g

This salsa is also good heated and served over sliced grilled steak or poultry.

Fiesta Salsa

4 fresh tomatoes, chopped
2 fresh green chilies, finely chopped
1 large onion, chopped
1 green bell pepper, seeded, stemmed, and chopped
1 tablespoon honey

1 tablespoon sherry vinegar
2 teaspoons olive oil
Salt and red pepper to taste
2 tablespoons chopped fresh cilantro
¼ teaspoon oregano

Mix together all the ingredients in a bowl and refrigerate.

 ## More About Salsas

Traditional salsa contains 3.2 grams of carbohydrates for a ¼-cup serving. Salsa Cruda is "uncooked salsa" made with fresh tomatoes, garlic, onions, and peppers. Salsa verde is "green salsa" made with tomatillos, green chilies, and cilantro.

Serves 2
Carb Level: Low
Per serving:
Carbohydrate: 9.9 g
Protein: 24.8 g

An easy dish for a large group. If you use frozen shrimp, make sure they are properly thawed before cooking.

Garlic Shrimp with Salsa

2 tablespoons extra-virgin olive oil
½ pound shrimp, peeled and deveined
Salt and pepper

1 clove garlic, minced
2 tablespoons salsa
½ avocado, sliced
½ jicama, shredded

1. Add the oil to a medium-size sauté pan over medium-high heat. Season the shrimp with salt and pepper; sauté for about 2 minutes. Add the garlic, turn the shrimp, and cook for another 2 minutes or until done.
2. Place the shrimp on warm plates and garnish with the salsa, avocado, and jicama.

Drunken Chicken

1 (4-pound) frying chicken, cut
    into 8 pieces
Salt and freshly ground black
    pepper to taste
1 teaspoon dried Mexican
    oregano
½ cup olive oil
1 large onion, thickly sliced

3 cloves garlic
1 bay leaf
½ cup dry white wine
½ cup tequila
1 cup Spanish olives, drained

<table>
<tr><td colspan="2">Serves 4</td></tr>
<tr><td colspan="2">Carb Level: Moderate</td></tr>
<tr><td colspan="2">Per serving:</td></tr>
<tr><td>Carbohydrate:</td><td>11.1 g</td></tr>
<tr><td>Protein:</td><td>81.4 g</td></tr>
</table>

This is a fun party dish
for a group of friends.

1. Preheat the oven to 375°.
2. Rinse the chicken under cold running water and pat dry with paper towels. Season the chicken with salt and pepper and oregano. Heat the olive oil in a large ovenproof sauté pan over medium-high heat. Brown the chicken pieces on all sides. Cook in batches if necessary to keep from overcrowding the pan.
3. Remove the chicken from the pan and set aside. Reduce the heat and add the onions and garlic; cook for about 5 minutes, until tender. Remove from the heat and add the bay leaf, wine, tequila, and olives. Return to the heat, bring to a simmer, and cook for about 5 minutes, until the alcohol is cooked off. Return the chicken to the pan, cover, and cook in the oven for about 45 minutes, until tender.

Mexican Cheeses

Authentic Mexican cheeses really enhance your south-of-the-border entrées. Good melting cheeses are Chihuahua and Quesadilla. Queso Cotija is a flavorful cheese used for grating or crumbling as a garnish. Cream-style Mexican cheeses include Cremma Mexicana, which is thicker than whipping cream and a flavorful addition where spicy chilies are used.

Pompano with Salsa Fresca

Serves 8
Carb Level: Moderate
Per serving:
Carbohydrate: 15.0 g
Protein: 24.0 g

Pompano have small scales that must be removed prior to cooking. Have your fish supplier do this for you.

4 cups diced plum or other ripe tomatoes
1 cup finely chopped Spanish onion
1 cup finely chopped cilantro
2 tablespoons chopped finger chili peppers
2 tablespoons extra-virgin olive oil
4 tablespoons fresh lime juice
2 medium avocados, peeled, seeded, and cut into a small dice
Salt and freshly ground black pepper to taste
8 pompano fillets
Olive oil

1. In a medium-size bowl, mix together the tomatoes, onion, cilantro, finger chilies, olive oil, lime juice, avocados, and salt and pepper. Allow to sit for about 1 hour at room temperature.
2. Preheat the broiler.
3. Coat the fish with olive oil and season with salt and pepper. Place the fish skin side up on a nonstick pan or baking sheet. Broil, about 4 inches from the heat source, until the skin is crisp and the flesh is opaque and white, about 6 to 8 minutes. Serve the fish, skin side down, with the prepared salsa fresca on top

Chipotle Chilies

Chipotles are actually dried, smoked jalapeños. Chipotles are hot and intense in flavor and are available dried or canned in adobo sauce. Adobo sauce is a vinegar-based sauce with ground chilies and herbs.

Guacamole

4 tomatillos, peeled, rinsed,
   and finely chopped
¼ medium onion, finely
   chopped
¼ cup coarsely chopped fresh
   cilantro
1–2 jalapeño peppers, seeded
   and finely chopped
1 clove garlic, minced

2 small avocados, peeled
   and pitted
1 tomato, cut into a small dice
1 tablespoon lime juice
Salt and freshly ground black
   pepper to taste

Serves 10
(makes 2½ cups)

Carb Level: Low

Per serving:

Carbohydrate:	5.3 g
Protein:	1.2 g

Use guacamole as a topping or accompaniment to grilled meats and poultry.

In a medium-size bowl, combine all the ingredients. Use the back of a fork to mash all of the ingredients until puréed but still slightly chunky. Best served the same day. Keep the avocado pit in the guacamole to prevent it from browning.

Substitutes for Seasonal Produce

You can substitute canned tomatoes and chilies if it's the dead of winter and quality vegetables aren't available. During the warm months, always use fresh, quality produce. There's no substitute for the flavor.

Mexican Tomato Salad

Serves 4
Carb Level: Low

Per serving:

Carbohydrate:	5.5 g
Protein:	1.6 g

Queso blanco (or queso fresco) is a white Mexican cheese, slightly salty, with a texture like Farmer's cheese

2 large, round ripe tomatoes, sliced ¼-inch thick
1 red onion, thinly sliced
2 serranos or jalapeños, thinly sliced
1 tablespoon chopped cilantro leaves
¼ cup queso blanco, crumbled
1 teaspoon Mexican oregano

1 teaspoon minced garlic
1 tablespoon extra-virgin olive oil
1 tablespoon white wine vinegar
Salt and freshly ground black pepper to taste

1. Arrange the sliced tomatoes, red onions, and chilies on a chilled platter. Sprinkle the cilantro and queso blanco over the top.
2. In a small bowl, combine the remaining ingredients. Drizzle the vinaigrette over the salad just before serving.

What Is Jicama?

Jicama is often referred to as the Mexican potato. It is a large bulbous root vegetable with a thin brown skin and white crunchy flesh. It has a sweet, nutty flavor that is good both raw and cooked. Fresh jicama can be added to salads for a satisfying crunchy texture. Jicama contains 3.8 grams of carbohydrates per ⅓ cup.

Roasted Pork with Asian Glaze ❖	80
Grilled Swordfish with Wasabi and Spinach	81
Shrimp with Plum Dipping Sauce ❖	82
Red Snapper with Garlic Ginger Sauce	83
Szechuan Shrimp with Chili Sauce	84
Asian Broccoli	85
Coconut Chicken ❖	86
Grilled Beef Tenderloin with Shiitake Sauce	87
Chicken Skewers with Spicy Island Marinade	88
Sea Scallops with Ginger Sauce	89
Cod with Lemongrass Sauce	90
Thai Vinaigrette ❖	91
Thai Beef Salad ❖	92
Grilled Tuna with Asian Slaw	93

❖ Indicates Easy Recipe ❖

Roasted Pork
with Asian Glaze

Serves 6
Carb Level: Low

Per serving:

Carbohydrate:	5.3 g
Protein:	26.5 g

You can let the meat marinate for up to 8 to 10 hours. Pair it with an assortment of Asian vegetables.

ॐ

2 pounds boneless fresh pork butt, loin, or shoulder
3 tablespoons soy sauce
3 tablespoons dry sherry
2 tablespoons Chinese barbecue sauce
1 tablespoon sugar
3 tablespoons peanut oil
1 teaspoon salt
1/4 teaspoon freshly ground white pepper

1. Cut the pork into strips, about 3/4-inch thick and about 1 1/2 inches long. Trim off any excess fat. In a medium-size bowl, mix together the remaining ingredients. Add the pork to the marinade, mixing to ensure the meat is evenly coated. Let stand, refrigerated and uncovered, for about 4 hours.

2. Preheat the oven to 400°.

3. Place the pork in an oiled baking dish and roast, uncovered, for about 30 minutes, turning several times. Make a tent with tin foil to cover the meat during the last 15 to 20 minutes of cooking if it appears to be browning too quickly. Let rest for about 5 minutes to allow the juices to absorb and serve hot. Can be used as a filling or served with a side salad.

Grilled Swordfish
with Wasabi and Spinach

1½ teaspoons wasabi powder
1 tablespoon water
1 tablespoon sesame seeds
1 pound fresh baby spinach
  leaves
2 tablespoons soy sauce or
  tamari, divided
Juice of ½ lemon
4 (1-inch-thick) swordfish steaks
  (about 6 ounces each)

Salt and freshly ground black
  pepper to taste
Juice of ½ lime
2 scallions, white and green
  parts, finely minced

Serves 4
Carb Level: Low

Per serving:

Carbohydrate:	6.2 g
Protein:	38.0 g

You can use frozen spinach as a time-saving step. Wasabi powder is available in Asian markets.

1. Prepare a charcoal grill or preheat a gas grill to very hot.
2. Set a large pot of salted water to boil. In a small bowl, mix the wasabi powder with 1 tablespoon of water and set aside.
3. Toast the sesame seeds, dry, in a small sauté pan over low heat, shaking them occasionally to brown them evenly. This will take about 3 to 4 minutes.
4. When the water comes to a boil, plunge the spinach into it and cook for only about 1 minute. Transfer the spinach to a bowl of ice water. Drain the spinach and use your hands to squeeze out any remaining water. Chop the spinach, then mix it with 1 tablespoon of the soy sauce, the lemon juice, and half of the sesame seeds; set aside.
5. Using a knife or a small spatula, spread the wasabi paste onto the swordfish. Season each side with salt and pepper. Grill the steaks for about 4 minutes on each side or until done. To check for doneness, use a thin-bladed knife to check between the layers of flesh to ensure no translucence remains and the meat is flaky. To serve, lay the fish on top of the spinach. Drizzle with the remaining soy sauce and lime juice. Garnish with the rest of the sesame seeds and the minced scallions.

Shrimp
with Plum Dipping Sauce

Serves 6
Carb Level: Low

Per serving:

Carbohydrate:	9.1 g
Protein:	15.9 g

Serve the shrimp on petite skewers for a fun party dish. You can also substitute strips of boneless sautéed chicken breast for the shrimp.

3 ripe plums, pits removed, peeled, and cut into pieces
1 cup water
½ teaspoon minced fresh ginger
3 tablespoons rice vinegar
1½ teaspoons Chinese five-spice powder
1 teaspoon chopped jalapeño pepper

2 tablespoons olive oil
1 pound shrimp, peeled and deveined
Salt and freshly ground black pepper

1. Place the plums in a blender. Add the water and process at high speed until puréed. Pour the purée into a medium-size saucepan and add the ginger, rice vinegar, five-spice powder, and jalapeño. Simmer over low heat, uncovered, for 20 minutes to reduce and thicken the sauce. Stir frequently to prevent scorching. Adjust seasoning to taste.
2. Add the oil to a medium-size sauté pan over medium-high heat. Season the shrimp with salt and pepper. Cook the shrimp for about 2 minutes on each side, until done. Serve on a warmed platter with the warm dipping sauce.

More about Rice Wine

The most popular types of rice wine used in the United States are mirin and sake. Mirin makes a flavorful base for Asian sauces.

Red Snapper
with Garlic Ginger Sauce

¾ cup vegetable oil
2 (1–1½ pound total)
  whole red snappers,
  cleaned, scaled, and patted
  dry on paper towels
2 tablespoons peanut oil
1 tablespoon minced garlic
1 teaspoon peeled and minced
  fresh ginger

1 tablespoon soy sauce
1 teaspoon sesame oil
Minced cilantro for garnish

Serves 2
Carb Level: Low

Per serving:	
Carbohydrate:	4.1 g
Protein:	47.6 g

Cooking whole fish can be a challenge. This recipe is difficult to prepare for large groups.

∾

1. In a large nonstick sauté pan over medium heat, add the vegetable oil to a depth of ¼ inch. When the oil is hot, gently place the fish in the pan. (Be cautious of splattering oil.) Cook, uncovered and undisturbed, for about 8 minutes. Make sure you watch the temperature during the cooking process. The oil should be at a consistent heavy simmer. Monitor the temperature to ensure the oil does not get too hot and bubble over. Using tongs and a spatula, carefully turn the fish over and cook for about 7 to 8 minutes.

2. While the fish is cooking, heat a medium-size sauté pan over medium heat. Add the peanut oil to the pan. Add the garlic and ginger and cook until it just starts to turn golden. (Overcooked garlic will leave a bitter taste.) Add the soy sauce and the sesame oil; set aside and keep warm.

3. When the fish are ready, remove them carefully from the oil and allow to drain on paper towels. Serve the fish hot on a platter. Drizzle the sauce over the fish and garnish with the chopped cilantro.

Szechuan Shrimp with Chili Sauce

<table>
<tr><td>

Serves 4

Carb Level: Low

Per serving:

Carbohydrate:	8.8 g
Protein:	23.9 g

The assortment of chilies make this a spicy dish. You can adjust the temperature by using more or less chili paste.

</td></tr>
</table>

1 pound medium shrimp, peeled and deveined
Salt and freshly ground black pepper to taste
2 tablespoons hoisin sauce
2 teaspoons tamari
1–2 teaspoons chili paste with garlic (available in Asian markets)
½ teaspoon sesame oil
½ teaspoon hot chili oil
2 tablespoons ketchup
¼ cup rice wine
1 teaspoon fish sauce
½ teaspoon honey
3 cups peanut oil
2 tablespoons finely minced fresh gingerroot
½ cup minced scallions (about 4 large scallions, white and green parts)
3 dried red chilies
Fresh cilantro for garnish (optional)

1. Season the shrimp with salt and pepper.
2. In a medium-size bowl combine the hoisin sauce, tamari, chili paste, sesame oil, chili oil, ketchup, rice wine, fish sauce, and honey; set aside.
3. Bring the peanut oil to 375° in a wok.
4. Immerse half of the shrimp in the hot oil and cook for about 20 seconds or until just translucent. Using a slotted spoon, transfer the shrimp to paper towels; keep warm. Repeat with the remaining shrimp.
5. Drain all but 2 tablespoons of the oil from the wok. Over high heat, stir-fry the ginger, scallions, and the dried chilies for about 1 minute. Add the reserved shrimp and toss well to blend. Add the reserved sauce and stir to coat the shrimp. Transfer the shrimp to a platter or individual plates and garnish with cilantro.

Asian Broccoli

1 large bunch of broccoli

2 tablespoons peanut oil

5 large cloves garlic, finely
    minced

3 tablespoons peeled and finely
    minced fresh gingerroot

2 tablespoon light soy sauce

1 tablespoon rice vinegar

$\frac{1}{4}$ cup chicken stock

1 tablespoon sugar

1 teaspoon sesame oil

Serves 6
Carb Level: Low

Per serving:	
Carbohydrate:	7.0 g
Protein:	0.9 g

Make sure the broccoli does not overcook—it should be a vibrant green color when ready to serve.

1. Cut the broccoli into small flowerets, keeping some of the stem on. Use a vegetable peeler to peel the tough part of the outer skin of the stems.
2. In a large pot of boiling salted water, cook the broccoli for about 2 minutes. Strain through a colander and run cold water over the broccoli to cool.
3. Heat the peanut oil in a wok or medium-sized sauté pan over medium heat. Cook the garlic and ginger for about 2 minutes, stirring constantly, being careful not to burn it. Add the broccoli, soy sauce, vinegar, chicken stock, and sugar; stir to blend. Remove the broccoli from the pan and set on a platter. Turn off the heat and swirl in the sesame oil; pour the sauce over the broccoli.

Add Tofu for a Meal

Using flavored pressed tofu is a quick entrée addition with stir-fried vegetables. There are a variety of flavors—including five-spice, teriyaki, sesame, and other Asian flavors—available in the Asian food section of the produce department in most supermarkets.

Coconut Chicken

Serves 4

Carb Level: Moderate

Per serving:

Carbohydrate:	18.3 g
Protein:	38.0 g

The natural sugars in the coconut milk and carrots bring up the carbohydrate level in this recipe.

∾

4 boneless, skinless chicken breast halves

1 tablespoon curry powder

2 tablespoons vegetable oil, divided

2 cups sliced asparagus, cut into 1-inch pieces on the bias

1 cup fresh snow peas

1 large carrot, peeled and shredded

4 green onions, green and white parts, sliced (about ½ cup)

1 (14-ounce) can coconut milk

1. Trim, rinse, and pat the chicken breasts dry with paper towels. Cut them into 1-inch cubes.
2. In a medium-sized bowl, mix the curry powder with 1 tablespoon of vegetable oil. Toss with the chicken pieces to ensure the meat is evenly coated.
3. In a large sauté pan over high heat, add the remaining tablespoon of oil. Cook the chicken in batches (to avoid overcrowding the pan) until golden brown, stirring frequently to prevent sticking. Return all of the chicken to the pan and add the asparagus, snow peas, carrots, and green onions. Cook for about 3 minutes over high heat, stirring constantly, until the vegetables are tender. Add the coconut milk and bring to a simmer. Serve immediately.

Low-Carb Substitutions

Yellow onions contain 3.5 grams of carbohydrates per ¼ cup. Substituting chopped scallions for the yellow onions changes the carb count to 1.8 grams—a reduction of almost half.

Grilled Beef Tenderloin
with Shiitake Sauce

*2 pounds beef tenderloin,
   trimmed of all fat*
*Salt and freshly ground black
   pepper to taste*
Olive oil
¼ cup unsalted butter
*1 tablespoon very finely minced
   fresh gingerroot*
*5 ounces fresh shitake mush-
   rooms*

1 cup heavy whipping cream
½ cup rice wine
2 tablespoons tamari
1 tablespoon honey
*¾ teaspoon grated orange
   zest*
½–1 teaspoon Asian chili paste
Fresh parsley for garnish

Serves 6
Carb Level: Moderate
Per serving:

Carbohydrate:	19.9 g
Protein:	30.4 g

You can substitute button mushrooms—which have a tenth of the carbs—for shiitakes, but don't expect the same flavor.

~

1. Prepare a charcoal grill or preheat a gas grill to 350°.
2. Season the beef with salt and pepper. Brush the grill with olive oil and grill the beef for about 30 to 40 minutes, turning about every 10 minutes, until the internal temperature of the meat reads 135° for medium-rare. Let the meat rest in a warm place for at least 10 minutes to allow the juices to reabsorb.
3. Place a large sauté pan over high heat. Add the butter and the ginger and cook, stirring frequently, for about 2 minutes. Add the mushrooms and cook until softened, about 3 to 4 minutes, stirring frequently. Add the whipping cream, rice wine, tamari, honey, orange zest, and chili paste; bring to a boil, stirring often, and reduce to a simmer until the sauce thickens.
4. Cut the meat into 4 even steak portions and place on heated plates. Spoon the sauce around the beef and garnish with chopped parsley.

Chicken Skewers
with Spicy Island Marinade

<table>
<tr><td>Serves 4</td></tr>
<tr><td>Carb Level: Moderate</td></tr>
<tr><td>Per serving:</td></tr>
<tr><td>Carbohydrate: 18.7 g</td></tr>
<tr><td>Protein: 36.1 g</td></tr>
</table>

This marinade may be made up to 3 days in advance and refrigerated until ready to use.

∾

Spicy Island Marinade:

¼ cup chopped scallions
¼ cup fresh lime juice
2 tablespoons chopped fresh parsley
½ teaspoon dried thyme
½ teaspoon dried crushed rosemary
1 teaspoon chopped garlic
1 fresh jalapeño, seeded and chopped
⅛ teaspoon (or to taste) hot sauce
Salt and freshly ground black pepper to taste

Chicken Skewers:

2 pieces boneless, skinless chicken breast (about 1 pound total)
8 white mushrooms, stems trimmed, and brushed clean
4 metal or bamboo skewers
Oil

1. For the marinade: Combine all the ingredients in a food processor and mix until finely chopped. Set aside until ready to use.
2. Slice each chicken breast into 4 equal pieces for a total of 8 pieces. Place the chicken in a plastic storage bag with a leak-proof seal. Pour the marinade over the chicken. Refrigerate for at least 3 hours.
3. Remove the chicken from the marinade. Discard the marinade. Thread a rolled-up strip of chicken on a skewer. Add a mushroom and another strip of chicken. Repeat with the remaining skewers.
4. Prepare a charcoal grill or preheat a gas grill to high heat. Lightly oil the grill rack. Grill the skewers on each side for about 5 minutes or until done. Turn the skewers several times to ensure all sides cook evenly. Transfer the skewers to a warm platter.

What Is Miso?

Miso is a concentrated bean paste that comes in three basic categories: barley, rice, and soybean. Miso is used in sauces, soups, marinades, and dressings. It is extremely nutritious—rich in B vitamins and high in protein. Miso is becoming more readily available in the refrigerator section of the Asian produce section of supermarkets.

Sea Scallops with Ginger Sauce

½ medium-sized leek
1 teaspoon unsalted butter
4 teaspoons olive oil, divided
3 shallots, minced
½ cup vegetable or chicken stock
¼ cup rice wine
3 tablespoons peeled and sliced fresh gingerroot
3 sprigs fresh parsley

4 sprigs fresh thyme
1 cup nonfat sour cream
1 teaspoon minced fresh gingerroot
Salt and freshly ground black pepper to taste
8 (1½- to 2-inch) sea scallops, trimmed of muscle and cut in half crosswise

Serves 4
Carb Level: Moderate
Per serving:
Carbohydrate: 17.4 g
Protein: 9.5 g

Scallops range in color from a light beige to a creamy pink; avoid ones that are stark white.

1. Trim the root end and the dark green top from the leek. Cut the white part in half lengthwise and wash thoroughly. Cut into thin strips.
2. Melt the butter and 1 teaspoon of the oil in a medium-size nonstick sauté pan over medium heat. When the butter is bubbling, add the sliced leeks and cook for about 3 minutes or until tender, stirring frequently. Remove from heat and keep warm.
3. Heat 2 teaspoons of oil over medium heat. Add the shallots and cook for about 2 minutes or until lightly browned. Add the stock, rice wine, sliced ginger, parsley, and thyme. Cook for about 5 minutes or until the liquid is reduced by half.
4. Strain the sauce through a sieve into a clean saucepan. Discard the solids. Place the pan over medium heat and whisk in the sour cream. Cook for about 3 minutes, whisking constantly, or until the sauce has reduced slightly. Add the minced ginger, salt, and pepper. Remove from the heat and keep warm.
5. Lightly brush a large nonstick sauté pan with the remaining 1 teaspoon oil and place over high heat. Season the dry scallops with salt and pepper. Cook the scallops in the hot pan, uncovered and undisturbed, for 1 to 2 minutes or until a golden brown crust has formed.
6. Using 4 small warm plates, place the sliced leeks in the center of the plates. Place the scallops around the leeks and spoon the sauce over the scallops.

Cod with Lemongrass Sauce

Serves 4
Carb Level: Moderate
Per serving:
Carbohydrate: 18.5 g
Protein: 35.5 g

Cod is an abundant, meaty fish. You can also substitute grouper, haddock, or red snapper.

ॐ

Lemongrass Sauce:

2 tablespoons extra-virgin olive oil
1 tablespoon minced garlic
1 tablespoon minced fresh ginger
4 tablespoons minced shallots
1 tablespoon chopped lemon-grass
4 tablespoons fresh lemon juice
2 cups chicken stock
4 large canned artichoke hearts, rinsed, halved lengthwise, and cut into very thin slices
2 tablespoons butter
Salt and freshly ground black pepper to taste

Cod:

4 (6-ounce) very fresh skinless cod fillets
1 teaspoon salt
2 teaspoons coarsely ground black pepper
2 tablespoons extra-virgin olive oil
Salt and freshly ground black pepper to taste
2 tablespoons chopped chives for garnish

1. For the lemongrass sauce: Heat the olive oil in a medium-size sauté pan over medium heat. Add the garlic, ginger, shallot, and lemongrass; cook until soft. Add the lemon juice and reduce by half. Add the chicken stock and reduce again by half. Purée the mixture in a blender or food processor. Add the artichokes and cook until heated through. Add the butter, and salt and pepper; keep warm.

2. Season the cod with the salt and pepper. Heat a large sauté pan over high heat. Add the oil and heat until very hot. Sear the cod for about 4 to 5 minutes on each side or until done. To check for doneness, insert a thin-bladed knife into the middle of the fish. All translucence should be gone and the flesh should be flaky. Transfer the fish onto a platter and spoon the sauce over the fillets. Garnish with the chopped chives.

Thai Vinaigrette

2 tablespoons hot chili oil
2 tablespoons sesame oil
¼ cup rice vinegar
Scant ¼ cup soy sauce

Whisk all the ingredients together. Shake well before using.

Vinaigrette—One of the Basic Sauces

This is a low-carb diet staple. In its simplest form, a vinaigrette classically contains 3 parts oil to 1 part vinegar seasoned with salt and pepper. This is used as a sauce for meat and fish, greens and vegetables. Variations include spices, mustards, citrus juices, herbs, shallots, and a variety of other flavorings.

Serves 4	
Carb Level: Low	
Per serving:	
Carbohydrate:	7.6 g
Protein:	7.6 g

Great over wheat noodles, salads, Asian vegetables, meat, and seafood. It can be refrigerated for up to 2 weeks.

Thai Beef Salad

Serves 4
Carb Level: Moderate
Per serving:
Carbohydrate: 12.3 g
Protein: 15.3 g

The steak and dressing may be prepared a day in advance. Thai Vinaigrette (page 91) also goes great over this salad.

ᔕ

Dressing:

4 tablespoons hot chili oil
4 tablespoons sesame oil
¼ cup rice wine vinegar
¼ cup soy sauce

Beef and salad:

1 (½-pound) fillet mignon,
    1–1½ inches thick
Salt and freshly ground black
    pepper to taste
Oil

4 firmly packed cups torn lettuce
    leaves
1 finely packed cup coarsely torn
    mint leaves, plus whole leaves
    for garnish
1 cup chopped cilantro leaves,
    plus whole leaves for garnish
½ cup purple basil leaves
1 cup thinly sliced red onion
½ firmly packed cup julienned
    daikon (white radish)
2 teaspoons finely minced fresh
    hot chili peppers
3 teaspoons fish sauce

1. For the dressing: Combine all the ingredients in a small bowl; set aside.
2. Prepare a charcoal grill or preheat a gas grill to high heat.
3. Season the beef with salt and pepper. Brush the grill with oil. Cook the fillet mignon for about 10 minutes on each side for rare. Allow the beef to rest on a plate tented with tin foil for at least 5 minutes.
4. While the beef is resting, combine the lettuce, mint, cilantro, basil, onion, daikon, and chilies in a large bowl.
5. Slice the beef into ⅛-inch-thick slices and toss them with the fish sauce. Add the beef to the bowl of lettuces, add the dressing, and toss. Serve on chilled plates and garnish with mint and cilantro leaves.

Fresh Ginger

Fresh ginger comes from a plant grown in Jamaica, India, Africa, and China. The flavor is peppery and slightly sweet, while the scent is spicy. Fresh unpeeled gingerroot can be stored, tightly wrapped, for up to 3 weeks in the refrigerator. The flavor of dried ground ginger is very different from fresh gingerroot and is not an appropriate substitute.

Grilled Tuna with Asian Slaw

2 tablespoons olive oil
½ teaspoon Thai chili sauce or
  other hot sauce
2 (1-inch-thick) ahi or yellowtail
  tuna steaks
Sunflower oil

Asian Slaw:

2 cups very thinly sliced red
  cabbage
2 cups very thinly sliced Napa
  cabbage
6 scallions, trimmed and slivered
  lengthwise

½ cup cooked green beans, slivered lengthwise
¼ large yellow bell pepper, cut
  into thin strips
Salt and freshly ground black
  pepper to taste
½ teaspoon toasted sesame oil
3 tablespoons sunflower oil
1 tablespoon rice wine vinegar
1 teaspoon soy sauce
1 tablespoon sesame seeds
2 teaspoons minced pickled
  ginger
1 small pinch of sugar substitute

Serves 2
Carb Level: Moderate

Per serving:	
Carbohydrate:	15.3 g
Protein:	43.6 g

Sushi-grade tuna is worth the extra expense. Ahi and yellowtail are the best tuna available.

1. Mix together the olive oil and the chili sauce, and rub it into both sides of the tuna.
2. For the slaw: In a large bowl, combine the red and Napa cabbage, scallions, green beans, peppers, and salt and, pepper. Whisk together the remaining slaw ingredients and pour over the vegetables; mix well to coat.
3. Prepare a charcoal grill or preheat a gas grill to high heat. Lightly oil the grill. Cook the tuna steaks for about 1 to 3 minutes on each side. The inside should still be rare. Serve the tuna steaks on top of the ginger slaw on a platter or individual plates.

CHAPTER 7

Salads and Dressings

Avocado and Cucumber Salad in Mint Dressing ❖	96
Chicken, Blue Cheese, and Apple Salad ❖	97
Spinach, Bacon, and Goat Cheese Salad ❖	98
Mushroom Custard with Blood Oranges and Crispy Greens	99
Greek Salad ❖	100
Fennel, Mushroom, and Parmesan Salad ❖	101
Roasted Beet Salad	102
Tomatoes with Green Goddess Dressing ❖	103
Mesclun and Fresh Herb Salad ❖	104
Caprese Salad ❖	104
Pears Wrapped in Prosciutto	105
Caesar Salad with Shrimp	106
Ham and Cheese Salad ❖	107
Lobster and Asparagus Salad	108
Ranch Dressing ❖	109
Blue Cheese Dressing ❖	109
Creamy Horseradish Dressing ❖	110
Balsamic Vinaigrette ❖	110
Orange Vinaigrette ❖	111
Sherry Vinaigrette ❖	111
Soy Sauce Vinaigrette ❖	112

❖ **Indicates Easy Recipe** ❖

Avocado and Cucumber Salad
in Mint Dressing

Serves 4

Carb Level: Moderate

Per serving:

Carbohydrate:	18.5 g
Protein:	6.8 g

Use English cucumbers for the best taste if the fresh garden variety is unavailable.

❧

Dressing:

¾ cup unpeeled cucumber
  slices
8 mint leaves
2 tablespoons chopped parsley
  leaves
2 cloves garlic, chopped
3 ounces firm tofu
4 tablespoons fresh lemon
  juice
1 teaspoon honey
Salt and freshly ground black
  pepper to taste

Salad:

1 head Boston lettuce, washed,
  patted dry, and cut into
  strips
2 ripe avocados, pitted, peeled,
  and sliced
1 cucumber, peeled and sliced

1. For the dressing: Combine all the ingredients in a blender or food processor and blend to a smooth, creamy consistency. Adjust with a little water if it is too thick.
2. Place the lettuce strips on a serving platter or individual plates. Arrange the avocado and cucumber on top. Drizzle the dressing over the salad and serve.

More about Avocados

Florida avocados contain about 30 percent less fat than the traditional Hass avocados.

Chicken, Blue Cheese, and Apple Salad

6 cups (about 8 ounces) packaged mixed salad greens or
mesclun
10–12 ounces roasted or grilled
chicken breast, sliced
¾ cup blue cheese dressing
2 ripe apples, cored and sliced

Freshly ground black pepper to
taste (optional)
Blue cheese crumbles for garnish (optional)

In a large mixing bowl, combine the salad greens, chicken, and dressing; toss gently to coat. Place on a large platter or divide among 4 individual salad plates. Arrange the apple slices on top of the salad. Sprinkle with freshly ground black pepper and blue cheese crumbles if desired.

Serves 4	
Carb Level: Moderate	
Per serving:	
Carbohydrate:	15.5 g
Protein:	31.1 g

Apples are a great source of vitamins A and C. Slice the apple just before serving to prevent browning.

ᘯ

Spinach, Bacon, and Goat Cheese Salad

Serves 2
Carb Level: Moderate

Per serving:

Carbohydrate:	18.8 g
Protein:	22.9 g

Be careful not to use too much dressing. The crisp saltiness of the bacon offsets the tang of the goat cheese.

∾

Dressing:

¼ cup light olive oil
2 tablespoons fresh lemon juice
1 teaspoon Dijon honey mustard
2 teaspoons minced fresh dill
Salt and freshly ground black pepper to taste

Salad:

¾ pound spinach leaves, washed
3 celery ribs, cut into thin 2-inch sticks
6 scallions, trimmed and slivered
2 ounces good-quality firm goat cheese, crumbled
½ cup sliced button mushrooms
4 strips smoked bacon, cooked and crumbled
2 tablespoons roasted sunflower seeds or soy nuts

1. For the dressing: Mix together all the dressing ingredients in a food processor or blender; process until smooth in texture. (Like most vinaigrettes, if the dressing sits, the oil and vinegar may separate; just stir again before use.)

2. In mixing bowl, combine the spinach, celery, scallions, goat cheese, and ¼ of the prepared salad dressing. Add additional dressing as desired. Toss to coat evenly. Place the salad on plates or a platter and sprinkle with the cooked bacon and roasted sunflower seeds.

Carb Facts for Vinegar

¼ cup of most vinegars contains 3.5 grams of carbohydrates. Balsamic, with its developed sugars, contains 3.9 grams of carbohydrates per ¼ cup.

Mushroom Custard
with Blood Oranges and Crispy Greens

2 ounces butter
4 shallots, chopped
1 pound mushrooms, sliced
*2 tablespoons chopped fresh
  parsley leaves*
Grating of fresh nutmeg
*Salt and freshly ground black
  pepper to taste*
½ cup heavy cream
4 eggs, beaten

Juice of 1 lemon
*3 cups mixed spring greens or
  herb salad greens*
*2 blood oranges, peeled and
  segmented*
*Chopped fresh herbs for
  garnish*

Serves 6
Carb Level: Moderate

Per serving:	
Carbohydrate:	18.2 g
Protein:	8.2 g

Button mushrooms have fewer carbs than others. Beware of using other varieties, as they will substantially increase the carb count.

∾

1. Melt the butter in a saucepan over medium heat and sauté the shallots, uncovered, until tender. Stir in the mushrooms, and cook until the mushrooms are tender, stirring frequently. Add the parsley and nutmeg. Season with salt and pepper, and allow to cool.
2. Preheat oven to 400°.
3. In a medium-size mixing bowl, beat together the cream, eggs, and lemon juice until smooth. Stir in the mushrooms and add a pinch of salt. Spoon the mixture into 6 greased ramekins, then place them in a deep rectangular casserole dish and fill the pan with boiling water to halfway up the sides of the filled ramekins. Bake for about 25 minutes, until the custard is set. Remove from oven and set aside to cool.
4. While the mushroom custards are cooling, place the greens on individual chilled salad plates and sprinkle with orange segments. Loosen the edges of the custards from the ramekins with a small, thin knife, then turn the custards over on top of the salad. Sprinkle with fresh chopped herbs and serve while still warm.

Greek Salad

Serves 2
Carb Level: Moderate

Per serving:

Carbohydrate:	14.7 g
Protein:	5.3 g

A great picnic treat. It is also very good after marinating overnight.

∾

½ ripe tomato, seeded
½ green bell pepper, cut into a medium dice
½ cucumber, peeled, seeded, and chopped
1 small sweet onion, cut into rings
1 clove garlic, minced
1 teaspoon chopped fresh dill
1 teaspoon dried oregano
3 ounces feta cheese, crumbled
2 tablespoons chopped fresh parsley
3 tablespoons extra-virgin olive oil
1 tablespoon red wine vinegar
Salt and freshly ground black pepper to taste

Place the first 9 ingredients in a mixing bowl. Mix the olive oil and vinegar together in a small bowl. Sprinkle a pinch of salt and pepper in the salad and toss with half of the dressing. Add more dressing as desired. Serve chilled or at room temperature.

Cheese Makes Everything Taste Better

Cheese makes a great topping for salads. Following is the carb and protein counts per ½ cup for the most popular cheeses:

	Carbohydrate	Protein
Cheddar	0.7 g	14.1 g
Colby	1.5 g	13.5 g
Cream cheese	3.0 g	8.6 g
Swiss	1.9 g	16.1 g
Blue cheese	1.3 g	12.1 g

Fennel, Mushroom, and Parmesan Salad

2 small (or 1 large tender)
very fresh fennel bulbs
Salt and freshly ground black
pepper to taste
3 to 4 tablespoons high-quality
extra-virgin olive oil
6–8 very large button
mushrooms, brushed clean

½ lemon
2 ounces good-quality
Parmesan cheese, at room
temperature

Serves 4
Carb Level: Moderate

Per serving:	
Carbohydrate:	10.4 g
Protein:	8.6 g

Use the best Parmesan and olive oil you can find. Baby fennel bulbs, if available, are excellent in this recipe.

∽

1. Remove any tough or bruised outer leaves from the fennel bulbs. Cut away the feathery tops and root ends. Wash the trimmed bulbs, and slice as thinly as possible (a mandolin, available at Asian food markets, is the best for this job). Layer the fennel over a platter. Season with salt and fresh pepper and drizzle with 1½ to 2 tablespoons of olive oil.

2. Slice the mushrooms as thinly as possible or shave the mushrooms on the mandolin slicer, producing almost transparent cross sections. Layer the mushrooms over the fennel. Top with a little more salt and pepper, a good squeeze of lemon juice, and the rest of the olive oil.

3. With a cheese slicer (or vegetable peeler), make about ¾ cup of parmesan shavings. Sprinkle the shavings on top of the fennel and mushrooms. Serve immediately.

Roasted Beet Salad

Serves 4
Carb Level: Moderate

Per serving:

Carbohydrate:	15.4 g
Protein:	1.8 g

Beets are a good source of vitamin A. This colorful salad is great for a brunch buffet.

1 pound unpeeled beets, washed and trimmed of green stems
3 tablespoons olive oil
1 tablespoon minced shallot
1 tablespoon fresh lemon juice
1½ tablespoons rice wine vinegar

1 teaspoon honey
½ teaspoon salt
3 cups (about 3 ounces) roughly chopped baby arugula
1 large apple, quartered, cored, and julienned

1. Preheat oven to 425°.
2. Wrap the whole beets in aluminum foil and roast in the middle of the oven until tender, 1 to 1½ hours. Unwrap beets and let cool.
3. While the beets are roasting, make the dressing by stirring together the oil, shallot, lemon juice, vinegar, honey, and salt in a large bowl.
4. Slip the skins from the beets and halve any large beets. (Wear plastic gloves while peeling and working with the beets, as they will stain your fingers.) Cut the beets into ¼-inch-thick slices and add to the dressing; toss to coat.
5. Arrange the beets on a platter and drizzle with any dressing remaining in the bowl. Top with the baby arugula, then the apple. Serve immediately.

Parmesan Cheese

Parmesan is a hard, dry cheese manufactured from skimmed or partially skimmed cow's milk. Parmigiano-Reggiano usually indicates the highest quality of imported Italian cheese and varies in aging up to 4 years. There are domestic pregrated Parmesan cheese on the market, but you should use the best wherever possible, as there is no comparison in taste and flavor. One ounce of fresh-grated parmesan packs in 41.6 grams of protein and 1.1 grams of carbohydrates.

Tomatoes with Green Goddess Dressing

1 cup mayonnaise
½ cup chopped fresh flat-leaf
  parsley
¼ cup chopped fresh chives
2 tablespoons chopped scallion
  greens
1½ teaspoons anchovy paste

1 teaspoon white wine vinegar
¼ teaspoon minced garlic
2 pounds medium beefsteak
  tomatoes

Serves 4
Carb Level: Moderate

Per serving:	
Carbohydrate:	10.7 g
Protein:	3.3 g

A simple and delicious addition to a buffet luncheon.

∽

1. Add all the ingredients *except* the tomatoes to the work bowl of a food processor (or a blender); purée until pale green and smooth. Transfer to a bowl and thin with a little water if desired.
2. Cut the tomatoes into wedges or ⅓-inch slices. Place the tomatoes on a platter or individual serving plates and sprinkle with salt and fresh ground black pepper. Drizzle the dressing over the tomatoes. Serve immediately.

 Dress Up Your Salad

The following garnishes are acceptable low-carb additions to dress up any salad presentation: crumbled crisp bacon, grated cheese, minced hard-boiled egg, and sautéed mushrooms.

Mesclun and Fresh Herb Salad

10 ounces mesclun (mixed
   baby lettuces)
½ cup fresh flat-leaf parsley
   leaves
¼ cup fresh mint leaves
¼ cup fresh tarragon leaves
¼ cup fresh basil leaves, torn
   into small pieces
Salt and freshly ground black
   pepper to taste

Toss together all the ingredients in a large bowl. Add any vinaigrette or dressing and toss again. Serve immediately.

Caprese Salad

1 cup extra-virgin olive oil
1 tablespoon red wine vinegar
1 teaspoon balsamic vinegar
⅛ teaspoon dried thyme
⅛ teaspoon dried basil
⅛ teaspoon dried chervil
1 teaspoon fresh chives
Salt and freshly ground black
   pepper to taste
Cayenne pepper to taste
¾ pound ripe plum or
   beefsteak tomatoes
20 fresh basil leaves
12 ounces fresh mozzarella,
   sliced into rounds

Combine the first 9 ingredients in food processor or blender; process until smooth. Slice the tomatoes into ⅓-inch-thick slices. Shingle the tomato slices, basil leaves, and mozzarella rounds in a circular pattern on a platter. Spoon the vinaigrette over the top and sprinkle with salt and pepper.

Pears Wrapped in Prosciutto

6 slices prosciutto
2 ripe pears
Extra-virgin olive oil
Salt and freshly ground black
*   pepper to taste*

4 cups mixed salad greens
Salad dressing of your choice
Fresh grated Parmesan cheese

Serves 4
Carb Level: Moderate

Per serving:	
Carbohydrate:	14.1 g
Protein:	23.5 g

Prosciutto is available at most deli counters. Use a good-quality Parmesan to enhance the flavors of this delicious salad.

℘

1. Cut each slice of prosciutto in half lengthwise. Cut each pear into 6 wedges and remove the core.
2. Toss the pear wedges in about 2 tablespoons of olive oil until evenly coated and season with salt and pepper. Heat a grill pan until very hot, almost smoking. Mark each side of the pear slices with dark brown grill marks on each side, using tongs to turn. This should take only a few minutes on each side. (If it takes longer, the pan needs to be hotter.)
3. Preheat broiler to low. Wrap a piece of prosciutto around the middle of each pear. Place all the wrapped pears on a lightly oiled baking sheet and cook for about 2 to 3 minutes on each side.
4. Serve hot on a bed of salad greens with your choice of salad dressing (vinaigrettes are best). Top the salad with Parmesan cheese, season with salt and pepper, drizzle with a little olive oil, and serve immediately.

Dressing Salads

Take care when dressing your salads. It's always easy to add a little more dressing but harder to remedy an overdressed salad. If you do use too much dressing, try adding more greens.

Caesar Salad with Shrimp

Serves 2 to 4

Carb Level: Low

Per serving:

Carbohydrate:	7.9 g
Protein:	29.3 g

Substitute grilled chicken or salmon for the shrimp if desired.

∾

Dressing:

1 tablespoon fresh lemon juice
1 egg yolk
Pinch of dry mustard
Salt and pepper to taste
Dash of Worcestershire sauce
2 cloves garlic, minced
½ inch squeeze of anchovy
*   paste from a tube*
*   (optional)*
6 tablespoons olive oil

Salad:

4 hearts of romaine, broken
*   into bite-size pieces*
2 tablespoons freshly grated
*   Parmesan cheese*
12 large shrimp, peeled,
*   deveined, cooked, and*
*   cooled*

1. For the dressing: Combine all the ingredients *except* the olive oil in a food processor (or blender). While the processor is on, slowly add the olive oil at a drizzle. Adjust seasoning to taste. (The dressing should be emulsified and will keep for up to a week.)
2. Put the romaine into a large bowl. Toss the greens with just enough dressing to coat the leaves. Sprinkle with the Parmesan. Dip the shrimp into a little of the dressing and arrange on top of the salad.

Health Hazards of Raw Eggs

This recipe contains raw egg yolk. Raw eggs can contain the bacteria salmonella, which can cause illness, especially in young children, elderly, those with health problems, and pregnant women. Though not common, you should consider this before consuming or serving products made with uncooked eggs.

Ham and Cheese Salad

1 (¼-inch-thick) slice ham
1 ounce Jarlsberg or Swiss
   cheese
½ cup sliced mushrooms
3 tablespoons chopped celery
2 tablespoons chopped parsley
1 tablespoon olive oil
1 teaspoon white wine vinegar
1 teaspoon Dijon mustard
1 tablespoon heavy cream

2 tablespoons freshly grated
   Parmesan cheese
Salt and freshly ground black
   pepper to taste

Serves 2
Carb Level: Low
Per serving:
Carbohydrate: 4.7 g
Protein: 18.8 g

A hearty entrée salad to be served well chilled either by itself, on top of lettuce greens, or rolled up wrap-style.

〜

1. Slice the ham into strips, about 2 inches long. Slice the cheese in the same manner. Put the ham and cheese into a large mixing bowl along with the sliced mushrooms, celery, and parsley.
2. Combine the remaining ingredients in a small mixing bowl; whisk together to blend. (You can add 1 to 2 packets of sugar substitute to make this more of a "honey" mustard dressing.) Adjust the salt and pepper to taste. Toss ¾ of the dressing with the ham and cheese mixture to coat evenly. Add more dressing if desired.

Don't Wash Those Greens (Yet)!

Salad greens should not be washed until just before serving. Loss of vitamins and minerals are increased as soon as the leaves are submerged in water. For best shelf life, store fresh greens wrapped in a damp towel in the crisper section of your refrigerator.

Lobster and Asparagus Salad

Serves 2
Carb Level: Low

Per serving:

Carbohydrate:	10.0 g
Protein:	34.5 g

You can ask your local fish market to cook the lobster and either keep it whole or shell the meat for you.

∾

Dressing:

1 small clove garlic, crushed
2 anchovies, well drained
1 tablespoon snipped fresh chives
1 tablespoon chopped fresh
    parsley
1 teaspoon chopped fresh tarragon
½ cup mayonnaise
1 teaspoon tarragon vinegar
Salt and freshly ground black
    pepper to taste
1–2 tablespoons sour cream
    (optional)

Salad:

1 pound asparagus spears
    (16–20 spears)
2 lobsters, claw and tail meat
    removed, shells discarded
2 cups mixed salad leaves
Fresh herb leaves for garnish

1. To make the dressing: Put the garlic, anchovies, and herbs in a food processor (or blender); process until smooth. Add the mayonnaise; process to mix. Add the vinegar, and salt and pepper to taste. Transfer to a bowl or other container, cover, and chill for at least 1 hour. Before serving, stir in a few tablespoons of sour cream, if desired, and adjust the seasoning to taste.

2. Trim off and discard the ends (1–2 inches) off the asparagus spears, making all the spears the same length. Use a vegetable peeler to peel off any tough outer layer on the stalks if necessary. Start about 1½ inches from the tip when peeling. Cook the asparagus in a pan of salted, boiling water for 4 to 8 minutes, depending on size, or until tender but still somewhat crisp and a vibrant green. Drain and rinse immediately under cold running water, then drain again. Leave to cool.

3. Slice the lobster tail meat into ½-inch rounds. Leave the claw meat intact. Arrange the asparagus spears and lobster meat on a bed of salad leaves on a chilled salad plate. Spoon a little of the dressing over the salad, garnish with the fresh herb leaves, and serve immediately.

Ranch Dressing

¾ cup buttermilk

2 tablespoons mayonnaise

2 tablespoons sour cream

½ tablespoon minced basil

1 tablespoon finely chopped
  fresh chives

2 teaspoons cider vinegar

1 teaspoon dry mustard

1 teaspoon fresh thyme leaves

1 clove garlic, minced

½ teaspoon sugar

Place all the ingredients in a blender or food processor and process until smooth. Adjust seasoning with salt and pepper to taste.

Makes 1 cup
Carb Level: Low

Per serving:	
Carbohydrate:	4.3 g
Protein:	2.1 g

Fresh herbs give this recipe a fresh clean flavor. Dressing will keep for 1 week covered and refrigerated.

Blue Cheese Dressing

½ cup sour cream

½ cup mayonnaise

2 scallions, minced

2–3 tablespoons fresh-squeezed
  lemon juice

½ cup blue cheese, crumbled

Freshly ground black pepper

Combine the sour cream, mayonnaise, scallions, and lemon juice in a bowl; mix well. Stir in the cheese and pepper. (The dressing should be salty enough from the cheese, but add a pinch if desired.) Cover and refrigerate for at least 4 hours before serving. The dressing will keep up to 5 days, covered tightly and refrigerated.

Makes 1½ cups
Carb Level: Low

Per serving:	
Carbohydrate:	3.0 g
Protein:	1.4 g

Process the ingredients in a food processor for a smooth creamy dressing, or mix by hand for a chunkier, country-style dressing.

Creamy Horseradish Dressing

Makes 2 cups

Carb Level: Low

Per serving:

Carbohydrate:	4.6 g
Protein:	29.9 g

This creamy salad dressing is also a great sauce for roasted salmon or steak.

²/₃ cup mayonnaise
1 cup sour cream
¹/₃ cup light whipping cream
5 tablespoons prepared horseradish

1 teaspoon Dijon or whole-grain mustard
Salt and freshly ground black pepper to taste

Whisk together all the ingredients in a mixing bowl. Adjust seasoning and horseradish to taste.

Balsamic Vinaigrette

Serves 4

Carb Level: Low

Per serving:

Carbohydrate:	1.8 g
Protein:	0.1 g

Add a little extra salt and freshly ground black pepper for a wonderful marinade for grilled vegetables.

¹/₃ cup balsamic vinegar
1 tablespoon minced shallot
1 teaspoon minced fresh marjoram or ¹/₂ teaspoon dried
1 tablespoon Dijon mustard

Salt and freshly ground pepper to taste
¹/₂ cup, plus 2 tablespoons good-quality extra-virgin olive oil

Combine all the ingredients *except* the olive oil in a mixing bowl; whisk to combine. While whisking, slowly add in the olive oil at a drizzle. Adjust seasoning to taste. Whisk before use if separated. This vinaigrette will keep 5 days, covered tightly and refrigerated.

Orange Vinaigrette

¼ cup champagne vinegar
3 tablespoons fresh-squeezed
orange juice
2 teaspoons grated orange rind

Salt and freshly ground black
pepper to taste
½ cup olive oil

Whisk together the vinegar, orange juice, zest, and a good pinch of salt and pepper in a mixing bowl. While whisking, slowly add in the olive oil at a drizzle. Adjust seasoning to taste. The vinaigrette will keep for 1 to 2 weeks in the refrigerator. Whisk before use if separated.

Serves 4
Carb Level: Low

Per serving:

Carbohydrate:	2.3 g
Protein:	0.1 g

This goes great with grilled chicken salads or as a sauce to accompany a grilled chicken entrée.

❧

Sherry Vinaigrette

⅓ cup light olive oil
⅓ cup walnut oil
1 teaspoon chopped shallot
½ cup sherry wine vinegar

Salt and freshly ground black
pepper to taste

Mix together the olive oil and walnut oil. Whisk together the shallot, vinegar, and salt and pepper in a bowl. While whisking, add the combined oil slowly at a drizzle. Adjust the seasoning to taste. Will keep for 1 to 2 weeks refrigerated. Whisk before using if separated.

Makes about 1 cup
Carb Level: Low

Per serving:

Carbohydrate:	1.9 g
Protein:	0.0 g

Walnut oil must be fresh and properly stored. Taste the oil before adding to ensure that it has not gone bad. Refrigerate after opening.

Soy Sauce Vinaigrette

Serves 4

Carb Level: Low

Per serving:

Carbohydrate:	2.5 g
Protein:	1.3 g

Mirin is a Japanese sweet wine used for cooking.

1 tablespoon sesame seeds
¼ cup rice vinegar
2 tablespoons mirin
2 tablespoons tamari or soy
  sauce

1 teaspoon sesame oil
  (optional)

1. Toast the sesame seeds (dry) in a small sauté pan over low heat, shaking the pan occasionally to toast evenly, until golden. While the seeds are still warm, crush them using a mortar and pestle (or with the flat part of a chef's knife).

2. Combine all the ingredients in a bowl and whisk to combine. Will keep for 1 to 2 weeks in the refrigerator; whisk before use if separated.

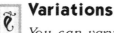 **Variations**

You can vary this recipe in several ways. Make it a little spicy by adding chili flakes. Add a teaspoon of freshly grated ginger and use it as a glaze for salmon. Or add two cloves of minced garlic and use it to season a simple stir-fry.

CHAPTER 8

Soups and Stews

Caribbean Shrimp Stew ❖	114
Bouillabaisse	115
Cream of Cauliflower Soup	116
Chicken and Mushroom Soup	117
Stilton and Cheddar Cheese Soup	118
Tomato Bisque ❖	119
Greek Chicken Lemon Soup ❖	119
Texas Chili	120
Onion Soup with Sherry ❖	121
Vegetable Curry Stew	122
Eggplant Stew	123
Herb Chicken Stew	124
Hearty Mushroom Soup ❖	125
Cold Fennel Soup ❖	126
Lamb Stew with Herbs de Provence	127
Red Cabbage Soup ❖	128

❖ **Indicates Easy Recipe** ❖

Caribbean Shrimp Stew

Serves 4
Carb Level: Moderate
Per serving:
Carbohydrate: 15.6 g
Protein: 25.4 g

A great dish for a casual get-together with friends for a summer afternoon party.

ℛ

1 pound shrimp, peeled and
  deveined
2 tablespoons fresh-squeezed
  lime juice
1/4 teaspoon ground cumin
Salt and freshly ground black
  pepper to taste
1 tablespoon olive oil
1 onion, finely chopped
1 small green bell pepper,
  finely chopped

1 small tomato, diced
3 cloves garlic, minced
3/4 teaspoon ground cumin,
  divided
1/2 cup tomato paste
1/2–3/4 cup dry white wine
1/2–3/4 cup lager beer
1 bay leaf
3 tablespoons finely chopped
  fresh cilantro or flat-leaf
  parsley

1. In a medium-size bowl, combine the shrimp, lime juice, cumin, and salt and pepper; stir to mix. Cover and marinate in the refrigerator for about 1 hour.
2. Heat the oil in a large nonstick sauté pan over medium heat. Add the onion, pepper, tomato, garlic, and 1/2 teaspoon of the cumin; cook for about 4 minutes or until lightly browned. Turn the heat to high and add the tomato paste; cook for about 1 minute, stirring constantly to keep the tomato paste from burning. Add 1/2 cup of the wine, 1/2 cup of the beer, and the bay leaf. Bring to a boil. Stir in the shrimp and reduce the heat to medium-low. Simmer for about 3 to 5 minutes or until the shrimp is cooked through. If the stew seems too dry, add more wine or beer.
3. Remove the bay leaf and season with salt and pepper. Serve in warm bowls garnished with chopped cilantro and a sprinkle of the remaining cumin.

Bouillabaisse

2 pounds mixed fish (cod,
   squid, salmon, etc.)
1 pound shellfish (shrimp,
   mussels, scallops, etc.)
6 cups water or bottled clam juice
1 medium onion, sliced
1 carrot, sliced
1 stalk celery, chopped
1 bay leaf
Salt and freshly ground black
   pepper to taste

2 tablespoons olive oil
2 cloves garlic, finely chopped
2 small leeks, trimmed and finely
   chopped
1 fresh fennel bulb, trimmed and
   cut into strips
4 tomatoes, peeled and chopped
3 strips orange peel, white pith
   removed
Good pinch of saffron threads
3 fresh thyme sprigs

Serves 6	
Carb Level: Moderate	
Per serving:	
Carbohydrate:	16.5 g
Protein:	32.0 g

You can make the vegetable broth a day early, then add the fish and shellfish to cook just before serving.

∾

1. Clean and prepare the fish. Remove the skin and bones and cut the fish into 2-inch pieces, but save any trimmings. (You can have your fish supplier do this step for you.) It is not necessary to peel the shells from the shrimp.

2. In a large saucepan, combine the fish trimmings and bones, water (or clam juice), onion, carrot, celery, and bay leaf. Bring to just a simmer and season with salt and pepper. Skim off any impurities that rise to the top, and simmer for 30 minutes. Strain the stock into a large bowl, discarding the bones and vegetables; set aside.

3. Add the oil to a large saucepan over medium heat. Cook the garlic, leeks, and fennel for about 5 minutes, until tender. Add the tomatoes and cook an additional 5 minutes. Pour in the reserved fish stock and bring to a simmer. Stir in the orange peel, saffron, and thyme; bring to a simmer. Add the mixed fish to the saucepan and simmer for about 8 minutes. Then add the shellfish and cook for 5 minutes. The mussels are cooked when the shells are completely opened. Season with salt and pepper and serve.

Cream of Cauliflower Soup

Serves 6
Carb Level: Moderate

Per serving:	
Carbohydrate:	11.6 g
Protein:	5.4 g

The cheese toasts do increase the carbohydrate count in this recipe. They are a nice touch but can easily be omitted.

ᔕ

1 large head cauliflower
¼ cup butter
1 medium onion, chopped
2 cups chicken stock
2 cups milk
Salt and freshly ground black
    pepper to taste
Pinch of nutmeg
¼ cup crème fraîche or sour
    cream

Cheese diamonds:

2 tablespoons grated Parmesan
    cheese
3 tablespoons butter, softened
2 medium-size slices of bread,
    crusts removed

1. Cut the cauliflower into flowerets. In a large pot of boiling salted water, blanch the cauliflower for 3 minutes. Drain through a colander.
2. Melt the butter in a large saucepan over medium heat. Add the onion and cook until tender. Add the stock, bring to a boil; and reduce to a simmer for about 20 minutes. Stir in the milk and add the cauliflower. Season with salt and pepper. Add nutmeg and simmer for 10 minutes. Using a slotted spoon, remove and reserve ⅓ of the cauliflower.
3. In a blender or food processor, blend the soup until smooth. Strain the soup through a fine-mesh sieve into a clean saucepan. Stir in the crème fraîche (*or* sour cream) and add the reserved cauliflower. Reheat very gently.
4. For the cheese diamonds: Preheat the oven to 400°.
5. Mix the cheese and butter in a small bowl until smooth. Spread this mixture over the bread. (You can use any type of bread.) Cut into small squares or diamonds. Place on a baking sheet and bake until golden brown. Serve alongside soup.

Cauliflower

Cauliflower is frequently used as a substitute for potatoes in low-carb cooking. Look for heads that are white or creamy white, firm, and compact.

Chicken and Mushroom Soup

1 bouquet garni:
   1 bay leaf
   ¼ teaspoon thyme
   3 sprigs parsley
1 (4–5 pound) chicken, cut
   into 8 pieces
2 medium onions, quartered
2 peeled carrots, coarsely
   chopped
1 cup celery, chopped
1 tablespoon butter

¼ pound button mushrooms,
   thinly sliced
Salt and freshly ground black
   pepper to taste
2 teaspoons fresh-squeezed
   lemon juice
½ cup chopped fresh parsley

Serves 6
Carb Level: Moderate

Per serving:	
Carbohydrate:	14.4 g
Protein:	44.7 g

Make a large batch and freeze individual portions to enjoy later or to give to a friend who is feeling under the weather.

1. To prepare the bouquet garni, wrap the bay leaf, thyme, and parsley in cheesecloth and tie with a string to create a little bundle.
2. In a medium-size saucepan, combine the chicken, onions, carrots, celery, and bouquet garni. Add water to cover and bring to a simmer. Skim off any impurities that rise to the top. Simmer, uncovered, until the chicken is tender, about 2 hours.
3. Remove the chicken from the saucepan and pull the meat from the bones. Cut the white meat into a small dice and set aside. This should yield about 1½ to 2 cups. (Discard the dark meat, or save it for another use). Strain the stock through a fine-mesh sieve into a bowl; discard the vegetables; set the meat and stock aside.
4. Add the butter to a medium-size saucepan over medium heat. When the butter begins to bubble, add the mushrooms and cook until tender. Season with salt and pepper. Add the reserved chicken stock, bring to a simmer, and cook for about 10 minutes. Add the lemon juice and the fresh parsley to finish the soup. Serve in warm bowls and garnish with the diced chicken meat.

Stilton and Cheddar Cheese Soup

Serves 8
Carb Level: Low

Per serving:

Carbohydrate:	2.8 g
Protein:	13.5 g

A very rich soup that goes perfectly with a salad for a full winter meal.

∾

2 tablespoons butter
½ cup finely chopped onion
½ cup finely chopped, peeled carrot
½ cup finely chopped celery
1 teaspoon finely minced garlic
3 cups chicken stock
½ cup crumbled Stilton cheese
½ cup diced Cheddar cheese
⅛ teaspoon baking soda
1 cup heavy cream

⅓ cup dry white wine
Salt and freshly ground black pepper to taste
Dash of cayenne pepper
1 bay leaf
¼ cup chopped fresh parsley for garnish

1. Melt the butter in a large saucepan over medium-high heat. Add the onion, carrot, celery, and garlic; sauté for about 8 minutes or until soft.
2. Add the stock, cheeses, baking soda, cream, wine, bay leaf, salt, pepper, and cayenne pepper. Stir well to combine. Bring to a boil, reduce the heat to low, and simmer for about 10 minutes. Remove the bay leaf. In a food processor or blender, purée the soup until smooth. Add milk to the soup if it is too thick.
3. Serve in warm soup bowls and garnish with fresh parsley.

Tomato Bisque

2 pounds ripe tomatoes, chopped
3 green onions, chopped
½ red bell pepper, seeded and
    chopped
2 cloves garlic, crushed
2 cups chicken stock

1 teaspoon sugar
¼ cup plain yogurt
2 tablespoons chopped fresh basil
Salt and freshly ground black
    pepper to taste
Chopped chives for garnish

1. In a large saucepan, combine the tomatoes, green onions, red pepper, garlic, stock, and sugar; bring to a boil, reduce to a simmer, and cook for about 15 minutes. Remove from the heat and let cool.
2. In a blender or a food processor, purée the soup until smooth. Strain the soup through a fine-mesh sieve into a bowl. Cover and refrigerate until chilled. Stir in the yogurt, basil, and salt and pepper. Serve in chilled bowls garnished with chopped chives.

Serves 6
Carb Level: Moderate

Per serving:	
Carbohydrate:	13.8 g
Protein:	3.0 g

This is a wonderful summer soup that is best served chilled. It is a great accompaniment to grilled chicken and a salad.

Greek Chicken Lemon Soup

4 cups chicken stock
4 eggs
4 tablespoons fresh lemon juice
½ cup whipping cream, whipped
    to soft peaks (optional)

Thin slices of whole lemon,
    seeded, for garnish

1. In a medium-size saucepan, bring the chicken stock to a boil.
2. In a small bowl, beat the eggs with a whisk until they are frothy, then add the lemon juice.
3. Slowly ladle 2 cups of the hot chicken stock into the egg mixture, whisking constantly. Pour the egg mixture back into the remaining stock, whisking over low heat until the soup thickens. This will take about 4 minutes. Serve in warm bowls garnished with a dollop of whipping cream and a slice of lemon.

Serves 4
Carb Level: Low

Per serving:	
Carbohydrate:	6.6 g
Protein:	8.1 g

Skip the whipped cream if you want a light creamy soup to accompany a heavier meal.

Texas Chili

Serves 2
Carb Level: Moderate
Per serving:
Carbohydrate: 11.8 g
Protein: 55.6 g

You can double this recipe and freeze individual portions for later use.

～

2 tablespoons vegetable oil
1 pound beef sirloin, coarse grind
½ cup chopped onion
3 cloves garlic, minced
2 tablespoons chili powder
½ teaspoon crushed dried oregano
½ teaspoon paprika
½ teaspoon dried cumin
½ teaspoon ground cumin
¼ teaspoon cayenne pepper
¼ cup tomato purée
½ cup diced tomatoes, with juice
½ cup beef broth
3 tablespoons grated Cheddar cheese

1. Heat the oil in a large sauté pan over medium-high heat. Add the beef and cook, uncovered, until browned. Add the onion, garlic, and all of the dried seasonings; stir well to mix, and cook until the onions are tender.
2. Transfer to a saucepan with a cover and add the tomato purée, diced tomatoes, and the broth. Simmer, covered, for about 1 hour, adding a little water or additional beef stock if the mixture appears too dry: it should be thick and soupy. Serve in warm bowls garnished with grated Cheddar cheese.

Onion Soup with Sherry

4 ounces butter
1 pound onions, thinly sliced
¼ cup whole wheat flour
½ cup dry sherry
6 cups chicken stock
1 cup grated Gruyère cheese,
   plus extra for garnish
1 tablespoon salt

Freshly ground black pepper
Large pinch of dried thyme
Large pinch of dried mace

Serves 6

Carb Level: Low

Per serving:	
Carbohydrate:	7.0 g
Protein:	4.0 g

Beware of chicken stock with too much salt (which will ruin the flavor). Look for homemade frozen stocks at local delis, or make your own.

Heat the butter in a large saucepan over medium heat. Cook the onions for about 6 minutes or until tender. Sprinkle in the flour and stir well. Stir in the sherry and stock, and simmer for about 20 minutes. Add the cheese, salt, pepper, thyme, and mace. Simmer for another 5 minutes. Serve in warm bowls garnished with grated cheese.

Recognizing Fresh Mussels and Clams
A good rule of thumb to follow when preparing shellfish is to throw away any mussels or clams that remain open when raw and any that remain closed when cooked.

Vegetable Curry Stew

Serves 8
Carb Level: Moderate

Per serving:

Carbohydrate:	18.1 g
Protein:	3.4 g

Top each portion of the stew with a piece of grilled chicken for a complete entrée.

❧

6 tablespoons olive oil
2 cups diced onions
1 red bell pepper, diced
6 tablespoons curry powder
2 tablespoons garlic, chopped
2 tablespoons peeled and
    minced fresh ginger
Salt and freshly ground black
    pepper to taste
2 cups large-diced pumpkin
2 chayote, peeled, seeded, and
    coarsely chopped
2 cups diced carrots
6 sprigs thyme
1 cup chopped scallions
Chicken stock or water to cover
1 head cauliflower, cut into
    florets

1. Put the oil in a large heavy-bottomed braising pot, with a cover, over medium-high heat. Cook the onions for about 2 minutes or until tender. Add the pepper and cook for another 2 minutes. Add the curry powder and sauté until fragrant. Add the garlic, ginger, and salt and pepper; cook for about 2 minutes.
2. Add the pumpkin, chayote, carrots, thyme, and scallions; cook for about 6 minutes. Add the stock (or water) to cover and bring to a simmer. Add the cauliflower and cover the pot; simmer for about 35 minutes. Add salt and pepper to taste.

Is Your Store-Bought Broth Low-Carb?

Premade stock and broths are available in tetra packs, canned, frozen, or concentrated. Note the "average" carbohydrate counts for a 1-cup serving of the following stocks:

Chicken stock	0.9 g
Beef stock	0.8 g
Vegetable stock	32.6 g

Eggplant Stew

4 whole eggplants, cut in half
Olive oil
Salt and freshly ground black
    pepper to taste
1 Spanish onion, chopped
4 cloves garlic, chopped

2 round ripe tomatoes,
    chopped
1 teaspoon hot pepper sauce
1 tablespoon ketchup
1 tablespoon chopped fresh
    parsley for garnish

1. Preheat the oven to 400°.
2. Brush the eggplants with olive oil and season them with salt and pepper. Roast the eggplants in the oven on a nonstick baking sheet, turning occasionally until soft, about 45 minutes. Remove from the oven and allow to cool.
3. Use a spoon to scoop out the flesh of the eggplant. Reserve the flesh and discard the skins.
4. Add 2 tablespoons of oil to a large sauté pan over medium heat. Add the onion and garlic; cook until tender, stirring frequently. Add the eggplant meat, tomatoes, hot pepper sauce, and, ketchup. Serve at room temperature in individual ramekins and garnish with chopped parsley.

Serves 8	
Carb Level: Moderate	
Per serving:	
Carbohydrate:	18.2 g
Protein:	3.0 g

Serve in preheated ramekins for a great starter course. Use eggplants that are firm, smooth-skinned, and even in color.

Herb Chicken Stew

Serves 6

Carb Level: Low

Per serving:	
Carbohydrate:	9.9 g
Protein:	30.1 g

Use any leftover chicken as a great filling for crepes.

2 pounds boneless, skinless chicken, cut into ½-inch cubes
1 tablespoon paprika
Salt and freshly ground black pepper to taste
Canola oil
2 onions, sliced
2 large carrots, peeled and cut into ⅛-inch slices
2 ribs celery, sliced
1 tablespoon dried thyme
2 tablespoons dried basil
1 tablespoon dried oregano
1 tablespoon ginger powder
1 tablespoon garlic
2 tablespoons soy sauce
1 quart chicken stock

1. Season the chicken with the paprika, and salt and pepper.
2. Heat 3 tablespoons of oil in a large heavy-bottomed stockpot over high heat; brown the chicken on all sides. (You may need to do this in batches to avoid overcrowding the pan.) Add more oil as needed. As the chicken is browned, remove with a slotted spoon and set aside.
3. In the same pot, add the onions, carrots, and celery; cook for about 6 minutes or until lightly brown. Season with salt and pepper. Add the thyme, basil, oregano, ginger, garlic, soy sauce, and stock; bring to a simmer. Return the chicken to the pan and simmer until the chicken is cooked through and the liquid is reduced by 20 percent. Season with salt and pepper.

The Benefits of Stew
Stewing not only tenderizes tougher pieces of meat, it allows the flavors of the ingredients to meld and develop in a way not attainable in short cooking methods.

Hearty Mushroom Soup

4 tablespoons butter
3 cups chopped mushrooms
½ cup chopped onions
2 cloves garlic, minced
Salt and cayenne pepper to
    taste
1 teaspoon dry mustard
2 teaspoons wild mushroom
    powder

3 cups chicken stock
2 tablespoons Madeira wine
¼ cup heavy cream, at room
    temperature

Serves 4
Carb Level: Low

Per serving:	
Carbohydrate:	5.2 g
Protein:	7.3 g

Grind dried wild mushrooms in a food processor to create the mushroom powder called for in this recipe.

1. Melt the butter in a large saucepan over medium-low heat. Cook the mushrooms, onions, and garlic for about 20 minutes or until the mixture seems thick. Add the salt, cayenne, dry mustard, and mushroom powder; mix well. Cook for about 5 minutes.
2. Pour in the chicken stock and Madeira; bring to a simmer. Allow the soup to cool slightly and then add the heavy cream very slowly, whisking constantly to ensure the cream does not separate or curdle. Return the pan to the heat and gently reheat, stirring until slightly thick. Serve immediately.

Save Some for Later

When making a batch of your favorites soup or stew, make an extra batch and freeze it to enjoy later. Your supermarket carries plastic freezer containers in ½-quart and 1-quart sizes, which are perfect for freezing. Always label the container with the contents and date. Soups and stews can be frozen for up to two months.

Cold Fennel Soup

Serves 6
Carb Level: Low

Per serving:

Carbohydrate:	9.4 g
Protein:	2.5 g

Fennel is a great source of vitamin A and contains a fair amount of calcium, phosphorus, and potassium.

∽

2 medium fennel bulbs
   (1 pound total)
1 tablespoon sunflower oil
1 small onion, chopped
3 cups chicken stock

Salt and freshly ground black
   pepper to taste
²⁄₃ cup sour cream

1. Cut off the green fronds from the fennel bulb and coarsely chop the bulbs and the fronds separately; set aside the chopped fronds.
2. Heat the oil in a large saucepan over medium heat. Add the fennel and the onion. Cover and simmer for about 10 minutes, stirring occasionally.
3. Add the stock and bring to a boil. Reduce the heat and simmer for about 20 minutes or until the fennel is tender.
4. Transfer the soup to a blender or a food processor; process until smooth. Season with salt and pepper. Strain through a five-mesh sieve into a bowl; chill in the refrigerator.
5. When chilled, whisk in the sour cream and adjust the seasoning to taste. Serve in chilled bowls. Garnish with the reserved fennel fronds.

Food Safety Tip

When reheating soups, always bring to a boil and allow to simmer for at least 3 minutes. This will effectively eliminate certain forms of bacteria that may have developed.

Lamb Stew with Herbs de Provence

2 pounds lamb fillet, shoulder,
   or leg
Salt and freshly ground black
   pepper to taste
2 tablespoons olive oil
½ cup chopped yellow onion
½ cup chopped carrots
1 tablespoon minced garlic

½ cup peeled, seeded, and
   chopped tomatoes
1 tablespoon Herbs de
   Provence
1 cup dry red wine
3 cups beef stock

Serves 4
Carb Level: Moderate

Per serving:	
Carbohydrate:	18.5 g
Protein:	32.7 g

Herbs de Provence is the most commonly used spice blend in southern France. It is available premade.

☙

1. Trim the fat off the lamb and cut the meat into 1-inch cubes. Season the meat with salt and pepper. In a large Dutch oven, heat the oil over medium-high heat. Add the lamb and cook until browned. (You may have to do this in batches to avoid overcrowding the pan.) Use a slotted spoon to remove the lamb and set aside.
2. Using the fat in the pan, add the onions and carrots, and cook for about 3 minutes until tender. Add the garlic and cook for 1 minute. Add the lamb, tomatoes, herbs, ½ teaspoon of salt, ¼ teaspoon pepper, red wine, and stock; bring to a boil. Reduce to a simmer and cook, covered, for about 45 minutes, until the lamb is tender. Serve in warm bowls.

How to Rehydrate Dried Mushrooms

Place the dried mushroom in a bowl and cover them with boiling water. Allow them to sit for at least 20 minutes and no longer than 40 minutes. The mushrooms should be soft, including the thick stem pieces. Drain the mushrooms, reserving the soaking liquid. Use the rehydrated mushrooms as called for in the recipe. Strain the soaking liquid to remove any grit or sand and add the mushroom liquid to soups, stews, or sauces for added flavor.

Red Cabbage Soup

Serves 6
Carb Level: Low

Per serving:	
Carbohydrate:	8.7 g
Protein:	2.5 g

Cabbage is a great source of vitamins A and C. This soup is based on the traditional Hungarian specialty soup.

ა

2 tablespoons olive oil
3 cups shredded red cabbage
1 medium onion, finely sliced
1 clove garlic, crushed
½ teaspoon caraway seeds
1 (14-ounce) can tomatoes, drained
1 tablespoon red wine vinegar
4 cups chicken stock
Salt and freshly ground black pepper to taste
¼ cup, plus 2 tablespoons sour cream
2 tablespoons chopped fresh dill
Fresh dill sprigs for garnish

1. Heat the oil in a large saucepan over medium heat. Add the cabbage and onion; cook, covered, for about 20 minutes or until the cabbage is soft. Stir in the garlic, caraway seeds, tomatoes, vinegar, and stock. Season with salt and pepper, and gently simmer for 30 minutes.
2. In a small bowl, combine the sour cream and chopped dill.
3. Serve the soup in warm bowls and garnish with a dollop of the dilled sour cream and dill sprigs.

Flavoring with a Bouquet Garni

A bouquet garni is a bunch of herbs—the classic being parsley, thyme, and bay leaf—that are either tied together or placed in a cheesecloth bag and used to flavor soups, stews, and broths. Tying or bagging the herbs allows for easy removal before the dish is served.

CHAPTER 9

Sides

Rapini with Chili Sauce ❖	130
Sicilian-Style Tomatoes ❖	131
Grilled Zucchini with Balsamic Vinegar ❖	132
Homemade Pickles ❖	133
Vegetable Casserole	134
Spinach-Wrapped Zucchini Flan	135
Sautéed Brussels Sprouts with Butter and Pecans ❖	136
Classic Coleslaw ❖	137
Collard Greens ❖	137
Grilled Radicchio with Fontina Cheese	138
Creamed Spinach ❖	138
Eggplant Timbale	139
Braised Fennel	140
Marinated Beefsteak Tomatoes ❖	141
Braised Baby Bok Choy ❖	142
Red Onions Braised with Sherry Vinegar ❖	143
Sautéed Mushrooms with Tarragon ❖	143
Sautéed Zucchini with Mustard Dill Sauce	144
Asparagus with Orange Herb Butter	145
Braised Savoy Cabbage ❖	145
Wild Mushrooms in a Brandy and Cream Sauce	146
Spiced Carrots ❖	147
Baked Garlic Tomatoes ❖	147
Garlic-Ginger Brussel Sprouts ❖	148
Zucchini Stuffed with Mushrooms	149
Turnip Gratin with Onion and Thyme	150

❖ **Indicates Easy Recipe** ❖

Rapini with Chili Sauce

Serves 6
Carb Level: Moderate
Per serving:
Carbohydrate: 12.1 g
Protein: 6.4 g

Goes great with pork dishes. You can find sweet chili sauce in Asian specialty markets.

❧

3 bunches broccoli rapini, trimmed, rinsed, and patted dry

3 tablespoons extra-virgin olive oil

4 cloves garlic, sliced paper thin

¼ cup Chinese sweet chili sauce

Salt and freshly ground black pepper to taste

1. Cut the rapini into large flowerets.
2. Bring a large pot of salted water to a boil. Cook the rapini for about 3 minutes or just until tender and a vibrant green. Drain through a colander and rinse under cool water. Set aside to drain.
3. Heat the olive oil in a large sauté pan over medium heat. Add the garlic and cook until soft, about 2 minutes. Add the rapini and cook, stirring often, until heated through. Toss in the sweet chili sauce and season with salt and pepper. Serve immediately.

Protein Facts

Protein-efficient foods contain 100 percent of the essential amino acids needed by the body. The most complete protein foods are eggs, fish, beef, whole cow's milk, and soybeans.

Sicilian-Style Tomatoes

4 firm, medium-size ripe
   tomatoes
Salt
4 anchovy fillets (optional)
2 tablespoons olive oil, plus
   extra for drizzling
¼ cup finely chopped onions
½ teaspoon finely chopped garlic
1 (7-ounce) can tuna (preferably Italian style, packed in
   olive oil), broken into small
   pieces

3 tablespoons finely chopped
   fresh flat-leaf parsley
2 tablespoons capers, thoroughly
   washed and drained
6 black olives, finely chopped
1 tablespoon freshly grated
   Parmesan cheese
Fresh parsley, finely chopped,
   for garnish

Serves 4
Carb Level: Low

Per serving:

Carbohydrate:	9.5 g
Protein:	15.7 g

The recipe can easily be doubled or tripled. You can also increase the number of servings by using small tomatoes.

1. Preheat oven to 375°.
2. Slice about ¼ inch off the top of each tomato. Using your index finger or a teaspoon, scoop out all of the pulp and seeds, leaving a hollow shell. Salt the insides of the tomatoes and turn them upside down over paper towels to drain.
3. Drain the anchovy fillets and soak them in cold water for 10 minutes. Pat the fillets dry, then finely chop them.
4. Heat the oil in a medium-sized sauté pan over medium heat. Add the onions and the garlic, and cook until soft but not yet beginning to color. Stir in the anchovy fillets and the tuna; cook for about 2 minutes, stirring often. Remove the sauté pan from the heat and add the chopped parsley, capers, and olives. Spoon the mixture into the hollowed tomatoes and sprinkle them with the Parmesan cheese and a few drops of olive oil.
5. Arrange the stuffed tomatoes in a lightly oiled baking dish. Bake for about 20 to 25 minutes, until they are tender and the cheese is golden brown. Serve them hot or at room temperature and garnish with chopped parsley.

Grilled Zucchini with Balsamic Vinegar

Serves 6
Carb Level: Low
Per serving:
Carbohydrate: 3.4 g
Protein: 1.1 g
This is a wonderful summer side to accompany grilled meats.

¼ cup extra-virgin olive oil
3 cloves garlic, finely chopped
4 medium zucchini, scrubbed and cut in half lengthwise
Salt and freshly ground black pepper
2 tablespoons balsamic vinegar

¼ cup coarsely chopped fresh herbs (mint, basil, chives, parsley, etc.)

1. Heat the oil in a small saucepan over low heat. Add the garlic and cook until just fragrant. Remove from the heat.
2. Prepare a charcoal grill or preheat a gas grill to high. Make sure the grill grate is clean and lightly oiled to prevent sticking.
3. Brush the zucchini with the garlic oil and season with salt and pepper. Grill the zucchini, skin side down, until it begins to soften, about 3 minutes. Turn, and cook the other side until tender; set aside.
4. Cut each piece of zucchini in half at an angle into 2 or 3 pieces and place in a bowl. Drizzle the vinegar over the zucchini and add the chopped herbs and the remaining garlic oil. Toss well and season with salt and pepper. Serve warm or at room temperature.

Homemade Pickles

1¾ cups cider vinegar
2 teaspoons pickling salt
½ teaspoon black peppercorns
½ teaspoon whole coriander seeds
2 Kirby cucumbers
1 small onion, halved and cut into thin slices

8 cloves garlic, crushed and peeled
¼ cup fresh dill sprigs, firmly packed

1. Bring the vinegar, salt, peppercorns, and coriander to a full boil in a medium-size saucepan over high heat. Cool completely.
2. Scrub the cucumbers, but do not peel them. Cut them into ¼-inch rounds or slice them into spears.
3. Sterilize a 1-quart jar by boiling it in water for 10 minutes or running it through a full dishwashing cycle. The jar should be hot when the vegetables are added.
4. Layer the cucumbers, onion, garlic, and dill in the hot jar. Pour in enough of the vinegar mixture to cover them completely. Screw on the lid and refrigerate for at least 3 days before eating. They will keep for up to 1 month in the refrigerator.

Serves 4	
Carb Level: Moderate	
Per serving:	
Carbohydrate:	19.8 g
Protein:	2.9 g

The longer the cucumbers have a chance to pickle, the better the flavor. This is a great picnic dish.

∾

Vegetable Casserole

Serves 6

Carb Level: Moderate

Per serving:

Carbohydrate:	19.5 g
Protein:	14.0 g

This is a great do-ahead recipe—bake partially the day before, then reheat and cook through when ready to serve.

4 tablespoons extra-virgin olive oil, divided
1 medium onion, chopped
2 cloves garlic, finely chopped
1 (15-ounce) can crushed tomatoes
1/4 cup chopped fresh basil
Salt and freshly ground black pepper to taste
1 medium eggplant, peeled and cut lengthwise into 3/4-inch-thick slices

3 medium zucchini, scrubbed and cut lengthwise into 1/2-inch-thick slices
2 medium-size red bell peppers, stemmed, seeded, and cut into 4 planks
8 ounces fresh mozzarella cheese, thinly sliced
1/3 cup dried breadcrumbs
1/3 cup freshly grated Parmesan cheese

1. Heat 2 tablespoons of the oil in a large sauté pan over medium heat. Add the onion and cook for about 5 minutes or until tender. Add the garlic and tomatoes and bring to a simmer. Simmer on low heat until thickened, about 10 minutes, stirring frequently. Add the basil, salt, and pepper; set aside.

2. Prepare a charcoal grill or preheat a gas grill to high. Make sure the grill grate is clean and lightly oiled to prevent sticking

3. Brush the sliced eggplant and zucchini with the remaining 2 tablespoons of oil, and place them on the grill. Add the red pepper planks to the grill, skin side down. Cook the peppers until the skin is charred, then remove them from the grill and peel off the skin. Return the peppers to the grill, cover, and cook for about 8 minutes or until all the vegetables are tender. Remove them from the grill and set aside.

4. Preheat the oven to 350°.

5. Lightly oil a 2-quart shallow baking dish. Spread a thin layer of the reserved tomato sauce in the bottom of the dish. Layer the vegetables, in any order, then the mozzarella, and the remaining tomato sauce, ending with a layer of vegetables. Mix together the breadcrumbs and the Parmesan cheese in a small bowl and sprinkle on top.

6. Bake for about 30 minutes or until the juices are bubbling and the top is golden brown. Let stand for at least 5 minutes before serving.

Spinach-Wrapped Zucchini Flan

1 large zucchini (about ¾
   pound), trimmed and cut
   into 2-inch pieces
4–6 large leaves flat-leaf
   spinach, washed thoroughly
   and stems removed
½ cup heavy cream
2 eggs
1 egg yolk

Salt and freshly ground black
   pepper to taste
Grating of fresh nutmeg
Tiny pinch of curry powder
Tiny pinch of cayenne powder
Butter, softened

Serves 4	
Carb Level: Low	
Per serving:	
Carbohydrate:	2.6 g
Protein:	2.8 g

The flan can be made
the day before and
gently reheated just
before serving.

∾

1. Preheat oven to 300°.
2. Bring salted water to a boil in a medium-sized saucepan. Using a steamer insert, steam the zucchini, covered, until tender. Add the spinach leaves to the steamer when the zucchini is just about done. When the leaves just start to wilt, remove them from the water. Spread them out flat on paper towels and pat dry. Remove the zucchini and let cool.
3. Squeeze the zucchini with your hands to remove as much water as possible. Transfer the zucchini to the work bowl of a food processor and process for about 30 seconds. Add the cream, eggs, egg yolk, salt and pepper, nutmeg, curry powder, and cayenne; process until very smooth.
4. Lightly butter four 4-ounce ramekins. Use the spinach to line each ramekin, positioning the leaves with the ribbed side facing inward. Leave a little spinach overhanging the edges of the ramekins.
5. Pour the custard into the spinach-lined ramekins. Fold the overhanging spinach leaves over the custard.
6. Place the ramekins in a baking dish. Fill the pan with boiling water ⅔ of the way up the sides of the ramekins. Bake for about 45 minutes or until just set. Remove the ramekins from the water and allow to rest for at least 5 minutes before unmolding.

Sautéed Brussels Sprouts with Butter and Pecans

Serves 4
Carb Level: Low

Per serving:

Carbohydrate:	6.7 g
Protein:	2.6 g

Take care to not overcook Brussels sprouts—they should remain a vibrant green with a bit of crunch.

1 pint fresh Brussels sprouts
3 tablespoons unsalted butter
½ cup roughly chopped pecans
¼ cup fresh-squeezed orange juice

Salt and freshly ground black pepper to taste

1. Bring salted water to a boil in a medium-size saucepan.
2. Trim off the ends of the sprouts and remove any bruised leaves. Boil the sprouts for about 5 to 10 minutes or until cooked through. (The larger the sprouts, the longer it will take.) Drain in a colander.
3. Cut each sprout in half. Heat the butter in a medium-sized sauté pan over high heat. When the butter just starts to foam, add the sprouts, pecans, orange juice, and salt and pepper. Stir until heated through and serve immediately.

A Tall Glass of Water

In the midst of counting carbohydrates, making sure vitamin and mineral requirements are in line, and ensuring an overall healthy diet plan, don't overlook the best low carbohydrate beverage available: Water! Water is a solvent and carries nutrients throughout your system to ensure each and every organ can do its job. Some dietary fiber and vitamins are water soluble, and water is the only way that your system can effectively absorb them.

Classic Coleslaw

2 cups mayonnaise
4 teaspoons sugar or sugar
    substitute
1½ teaspoons dry mustard
4 tablespoons white wine
    vinegar

8 cups shredded red or green
    cabbage
1 carrot, grated
1 onion, cut into a small dice
Salt and freshly ground black
    pepper to taste

In a large mixing bowl, whisk together the mayonnaise, sugar, mustard, and vinegar. Add the remaining ingredients, and mix well to coat. Refrigerate for at least 1 hour before serving.

Serves 10	
Carb Level: Low	
Per serving:	
Carbohydrate:	7.1 g
Protein:	1.6 g

Makes a perfect side dish for a picnic or a BBQ.

Collard Greens

3 strips slab bacon
1½–2 pounds collard greens
    (about 2 big bunches)
2 scallions, sliced

Salt and freshly ground black
    pepper to taste
Squeeze of fresh lemon juice

1. Cut the bacon into ½-inch pieces. Cook the bacon over medium-low heat in a medium-sized saucepot until the fat is rendered and the bacon is crisp.
2. While the bacon is cooking, cut off and discard the stems from the collard greens. Roughly chop the greens and wash them thoroughly.
3. Add the greens to the pot with the bacon, along with the scallions and 1 cup of water. Cover and cook over medium-low heat for about 2 hours, stirring occasionally. Add more water if it seems to be getting too dry. Season with salt and pepper and lemon juice.

Serves 6	
Carb Level: Low	
Per serving:	
Carbohydrate:	5.2 g
Protein:	2.1 g

This soul-food staple is an excellent source of vitamins A and C as well as calcium and iron.

Grilled Radicchio with Fontina Cheese

Serves 2
Carb Level: Low

Per serving:	
Carbohydrate:	3.0 g
Protein:	24.5 g

Fontina is a great Italian cow's milk cheese that melts easily and has a mild nutty flavor.

❧

1 large head radicchio
Olive oil
Salt and freshly ground black
    pepper to taste

2 (½-inch-thick) slices fontina
    cheese

1. Prepare a charcoal grill or preheat a gas grill to high. Make sure the grill grate is clean and lightly oiled to prevent sticking.
2. Trim off the stem of the radicchio and cut the head in half lengthwise. Brush the halves with olive oil and season with salt and pepper.
3. Grill the radicchio, cut-side down, until it starts to wilt and is slightly charred around the edges. Turn over the radicchio and top each half with a slice of cheese. (The cheese will melt as the other side cooks.) Serve immediately.

Creamed Spinach

Serves 4
Carb Level: Low

Per serving:	
Carbohydrate:	3.0 g
Protein:	1.8 g

This popular side dish can be prepared in advance; then reheated just before serving.

❧

1 teaspoon unsalted butter
1 teaspoon minced garlic
1 (10-ounce) package frozen
    spinach, thawed and mois-
    ture pressed out
¾ cup heavy cream

2 tablespoons chopped fresh
    thyme leaves
A few gratings of nutmeg
Small pinch of cayenne pepper
Salt and freshly ground black
    pepper
Squeeze of fresh lemon juice

In a medium-size nonreactive saucepan, melt the butter over medium heat. Add the garlic and cook for about 1 minute or until tender. (Be careful not to let it color.) Add the chopped spinach to the pot along with the heavy cream, thyme, nutmeg, cayenne, and salt and pepper. Cook over low heat, uncovered, stirring frequently until the cream has thickened and the spinach is very soft. Season with lemon and serve immediately.

Eggplant Timbale

1 medium eggplant, halved
Olive oil
Salt and freshly ground black
pepper to taste
½ cup milk
1 egg
1 egg yolk

Pinch of ground cumin (or to
taste)
Butter, softened

Serves 4
Carb Level: Low

Per serving:	
Carbohydrate:	8.6 g
Protein:	4.4 g

This dish is great with grilled meats and lamb dishes and works well with any entrée with Mediterranean spices and flavors.

1. Preheat the oven to 350°.
2. Brush the eggplant with olive oil and season with salt and pepper. Roast the eggplants in the oven on a nonstick baking sheet, turning occasionally, until soft. This will take about 45 minutes to 1 hour.
3. Allow to cool and use a spoon to scoop out the flesh of the eggplant. Reserve the flesh and discard the skins. In a food processor or blender, process the eggplant until smooth. Discard all but ½ cup of the purée (or freeze the extra purée for the next time you want to make this recipe). The frozen purée will last in an airtight container for 2 weeks. Add the milk, egg, egg yolk, salt, and pepper to taste, and cumin to the eggplant purée; process until smooth.
4. Lightly butter four 4-ounce ramekins. Pour the custard into the molds and place in a baking dish. Fill the dish with boiling water ⅔ of the way up the sides of the ramekins. Bake for about 1 hour or until just set. Unmold the custards and serve on the side with any main dish.

Vegetable Numbers

A ⅓-cup serving of the following vegetables contains few carbs:

Broccoli	*1.8 g*
Green beans	*2.6 g*
Zucchini	*1.3 g*

Braised Fennel

Serves 4	
Carb Level: Low	

Per serving:

Carbohydrate:	9.8 g
Protein:	1.8 g

A fennel lover's delight! This dish is relatively easy to pre-pare and is a perfect pairing with Italian-seasoned entrées.

2 large fennel bulbs
2 tablespoons olive oil
1 medium onion, chopped
1 cup chicken stock
1 teaspoon grated orange zest
1 teaspoon chopped fresh
   thyme
2 tablespoons Pernod (French
   anise-flavored cordial)

Salt and freshly ground black
   pepper to taste
2 teaspoons toasted anise
   seeds

1. Preheat oven to 375°.
2. Cut off and discard the leafy top of the fennel bulb. Trim off the base of the bulb and remove any brown outer layers. Cut the bulb in half lengthwise and trim out and discard the root core. Wash the fennel bulb halves and set aside.
3. Heat the oil in a large ovenproof sauté pan over medium-high heat. Add the onion and cook for about 2 minutes or until tender. Add the fennel bulbs to the pan, cut-side down, and cook for about 5 minutes or until they are lightly browned. Add the stock, orange zest, thyme, Pernod, and salt and pepper; bring to a simmer. Cover the pan and transfer it to the oven; bake for about 40 minutes or until the fennel bulbs are tender. Transfer to a serving dish and garnish with the toasted anise seeds.

More Vegetable Numbers
Carb counts per ⅓-cup serving:

Corn kernels	11.4 g
Peas	7.0 g
Asparagus	1.9 g

Marinated Beefsteak Tomatoes

*3 tablespoons aged balsamic
   vinegar*
*2 tablespoons extra-virgin
   olive oil*
*Salt and freshly ground black
   pepper to taste*
*1 tablespoon chopped fresh
   parsley*

*1 tablespoon chopped fresh
   basil*
*1 large ripe beefsteak tomato,
   cut into ½-inch slices*

Serves 2
Carb Level: Low

Per serving:	
Carbohydrate:	4.4 g
Protein:	0.6 g

Serve these tomatoes with just about any-thing—use as a garnish for burgers or serve with anything grilled.

In a medium-size bowl, whisk together the vinegar, olive oil, salt and pepper, parsley, and basil. Add the tomato slices and marinate for 1 hour before serving. Best served at room temperature.

 ## Choosing Tomatoes

Commercial tomatoes are grown more for shelf life than for flavor. It is better to substitute canned roma tomatoes for pulplike fresh tomatoes. The best tomatoes are fresh grown in your back yard or purchased from your local farmer's market.

Braised Baby Bok Choy

Serves 4
Carb Level: Low

Per serving:

Carbohydrate:	3.2 g
Protein:	1.6 g

Braising is a flavorful method for cooking most any vegetable.

~

4 heads baby bok choy
1 clove garlic, peeled and
   crushed
1 teaspoon Chinese 5-spice
   powder
2 scallions, thinly sliced

Salt and freshly ground black
   pepper
2 cups chicken stock

1. Rinse the bok choy under cold running water and pat dry with paper towels. Trim off the ends of the bok choy but be sure to leave the heads whole.
2. Place the bok choy in a large nonstick sauté pan along with all the remaining ingredients. Place the sauté pan over high heat and bring to a boil. Lower the heat to a simmer and cook for about 10 minutes or until the bok choy is tender but still slightly crisp.

Different Cooking Methods
Changing the cooking techniques of a recipe indicates a creative cook. Try poaching or steaming instead of sautéing or grilling. Experiment with your food and enjoy the cooking adventure.

Red Onions Braised with Sherry Vinegar

2 tablespoons chicken stock
1½ pounds red onions, peeled
   and sliced
2 teaspoons sugar

Salt and freshly ground black
   pepper to taste
3 tablespoons (or to taste)
   sherry wine vinegar

1. Heat the stock in a large saucepan over medium-high heat. Add the onions, sugar, and salt and pepper. Cook over low heat, covered, for about 35 minutes or until the onions are lightly browned.
2. Add the vinegar and cook for another 30 minutes, covered, over low heat. The onions should be very soft and glazed.

Serves 8
Carb Level: Low

Per serving:	
Carbohydrate:	8.8 g
Protein:	1.0 g

A perfect pairing with grilled meats or sausages.

❧

Sautéed Mushrooms with Tarragon

1 tablespoon olive oil
10 ounces button mushrooms,
   trimmed, cleaned, and cut
   into quarters
1 teaspoon minced garlic

Salt and freshly ground black
   pepper to taste
1 teaspoon coarsely chopped
   fresh tarragon
Squeeze of fresh lemon

1. Heat the olive oil in a medium-size sauté pan over medium-high heat. Add the mushrooms and cook them for about 5 minutes, stirring often, until they are lightly brown.
2. Lower the heat, add the garlic, and cook for 1 minute. Season with salt and pepper. Add the tarragon and a squeeze of lemon juice. Serve immediately.

Serves 2
Carb Level: Low

Per serving:	
Carbohydrate:	7.6 g
Protein:	2.8 g

This is a great side for seafood dishes.

❧

Sautéed Zucchini with Mustard Dill Sauce

3–4 whole zucchini
2 tablespoons olive oil
½ cup diced shallots or white onions
2 cups chicken stock
2 ounces half-and-half or cream
2 tablespoons grainy-style mustard
2 tablespoons Dijon mustard
½ teaspoon salt
½ teaspoon freshly ground black pepper
4 tablespoons chopped fresh dill, divided

1. Wash the zucchini and trim off the ends. Slice the zucchini into ¼- to ½-inch slices, to yield about 4 cups.
2. Heat the oil in a large nonstick sauté pan over medium-high heat. Cook the zucchini for about 1 minute on each side. Drain off any excess oil. Add all the remaining ingredients except the dill, cover, and reduce the heat to medium-low; cook for about 15 minutes or until the sauce has thickened and the zucchini is slightly soft.
3. Add 2 tablespoons of the dill and gently fold it into the sauce. Serve on a platter and garnish with the remaining chopped dill.

Asparagus with Orange Herb Butter

½ pound thin asparagus, tough ends trimmed off

4 tablespoons fresh-squeezed orange juice

3 tablespoons cold, unsalted butter, cut into small pieces

1 teaspoon orange zest, finely grated

Salt and freshly ground black pepper to taste

1 teaspoon chopped fresh chives

1. In a large pot of salted boiling water, cook the asparagus for about 1 minute or until just done. (They should be tender and a vibrant green.) Drain and arrange the asparagus on a platter; keep warm.
2. Heat the orange juice in a small sauté pan over medium heat until reduced by half. Take the pan off the heat and swirl in the butter a little bit at a time until the sauce thickens. Season the sauce with the orange zest, salt and pepper, and chopped chives. Pour the sauce over the asparagus and serve immediately.

Serves 2	
Carb Level: Low	
Per serving:	
Carbohydrate:	4.2 g
Protein:	1.7 g

If you can't find thin asparagus spears, just peel the woody stalks off thicker stalks with a vegetable peeler.

Braised Savoy Cabbage

2 strips lean bacon, cut into ¼-inch pieces

4 scallions, thinly sliced

6 cups shredded savoy cabbage

½ cup rice wine vinegar

1 cup chicken stock

Salt and freshly ground black pepper to taste

1. In a medium-size saucepan, cook the bacon over medium heat until the fat has rendered and the bacon is crispy.
2. Add the scallions and cook, stirring often, until they are soft, about 1 to 2 minutes. Add the cabbage, vinegar, and stock; mix well. Bring to a boil, then reduce the heat to a simmer. Cook, uncovered, for 15 minutes, stirring occasionally until the cabbage is soft but not falling apart. Serve immediately

Serves 4	
Carb Level: Low	
Per serving:	
Carbohydrate:	9.5 g
Protein:	2.6 g

Makes a great side dish with Asian entrées—or serve with grilled sausages for a traditional pairing.

Wild Mushrooms in a Brandy and Cream Sauce

Serves 2
Carb Level: Moderate

Per serving:	
Carbohydrate:	19.7 g
Protein:	9.6 g

This is truly an elegant dish and a great side for a simple entrée like grilled fillet mignon.

〜

3 cups raw mixed wild mushrooms
1 tablespoon unsalted butter
Salt and freshly ground black pepper to taste
1 tablespoon olive oil
½ teaspoon minced garlic
1 tablespoon minced shallot
2 tablespoons brandy
⅔ cup heavy cream

Squeeze of fresh lemon juice
Grating of fresh nutmeg
2 teaspoons chopped mixed light-flavored fresh herbs such as parsley, chives, and chervil (optional)

1. Trim off and discard the stems from the mushrooms. Clean the mushrooms with a damp paper towel or mushroom brush, then quarter them.
2. Heat the butter in a medium-size sauté pan over medium heat. Cook the mushrooms gently, stirring occasionally, for about 15 minutes or until soft. Season with salt and pepper. Remove from the pan and set aside.
3. Heat the oil in a medium-size sauté pan over high heat. Add the mushrooms and cook them until slightly browned. Add the garlic and shallot and cook for about 1 minute, stirring constantly. Be careful not to let the garlic and shallot color.
4. Remove the pan from the heat and add the brandy. The brandy will ignite, so be careful: stand back as you do this. Return the pan to the heat and cook until the brandy has almost evaporated. Add the cream, and salt and pepper, and reduce the cream over high heat until the sauce has thickened slightly. Add the lemon juice, the nutmeg, and the fresh herbs.

Spiced Carrots

1 pound carrots
1 cup vegetable stock
1 tablespoon honey
1 teaspoon ground cinnamon
½ teaspoon ground cumin
¼ teaspoon cayenne

½ cup fresh-squeezed orange juice
Grated zest of 1 orange
Salt and freshly ground black
   pepper to taste
Cayenne pepper to taste
3 tablespoons chopped fresh mint

1. Peel and slice the carrots about ¼-inch thick.
2. Bring the stock to boil in a large sauté pan over medium heat. Add the carrots, honey, and spices; stir well. Reduce the heat and simmer until the carrots are just tender, about 6 minutes. (They should remain a little crisp.)
3. Stir in the orange juice and zest, and simmer for an additional 2 minutes. Season with salt, pepper, and cayenne. Sprinkle with the chopped mint and serve.

Serves 4

Carb Level: Moderate

Per serving:

Carbohydrate:	19.2 g
Protein:	1.8 g

You can substitute frozen sliced carrots as a time-saving step.

Baked Garlic Tomatoes

½ cup fresh bread crumbs
½ bunch flat-leaf parsley, stems
   discarded, leaves chopped
2 cups frozen chopped broccoli,
   thawed and drained
¼ cup freshly grated Parmesan
   cheese
3 tablespoons heavy cream

20 basil leaves, chopped
4 cloves garlic, minced
1 teaspoon sugar
Salt and freshly ground black
   pepper to taste
8 tomatoes, tops cut off, seeds and
   juice removed, hollowed out but
   skin and meat should stay intact

1. Preheat oven to 325°.
2. In a medium-size bowl, mix all of the ingredients except the tomatoes. Stuff the tomatoes with this mixture.
3. Place the tomatoes in a baking dish and cook for about 45 minutes or until the tomatoes are soft and the tops are golden brown. Allow to cool for about 5 minutes before serving.

Serves 8

Carb Level: Moderate

Per serving:

Carbohydrate:	13.6 g
Protein:	6.5 g

This is a great stuffed vegetable for a dinner party.

Garlic-Ginger Brussels Sprouts

1 pound Brussels sprouts, ends trimmed

1½ cups chicken stock or water, divided

1 tablespoon finely minced garlic

1 tablespoon grated fresh gingerroot

1 teaspoon grated lemon zest

1½ teaspoons fennel seeds

Salt and freshly ground black pepper to taste

1. Cut the stems from the sprouts and remove any bruised leaves. Cut the sprouts in half and then into very thin strips.
2. Bring 1 cup of the stock (or water) to a boil in a large sauté pan. Reduce to a simmer, and add the sprouts, garlic, ginger, and the lemon zest. Cook, uncovered, over high heat, stirring often for about 5 minutes or until the sprouts are tender. Add the reserved stock if they are getting too dry. Stir in the fennel seeds and salt and pepper.

And Even More Vegetable Numbers

Carb counts for a ⅓-cup serving of each of the following vegetables:

Cauliflower	1.7 g
Fennel	2.1 g
Butternut squash	5.5 g

Zucchini Stuffed with Mushrooms

5 large zucchini, about 3
   pounds
6 cloves garlic, thinly sliced
12 ounces medium-size mushrooms, sliced thinly
1 yellow onion, thinly sliced
1 cup water
Salt and freshly ground black
   pepper to taste

2 tablespoons chopped fresh
   tarragon
½ cup peeled, seeded, and
   diced tomatoes
½ cup chervil leaves

Serves 4
Carb Level: Moderate

Per serving:

Carbohydrate:	15.6 g
Protein:	5.2 g

Zucchini should be vibrant in color and be blemish-free when you buy them. Fresh zucchini are available year-round in most supermarkets.

1. Trim the tops and bottoms from the zucchini. Cut 4 of the zucchini in half lengthwise and carefully scoop out the pulp and seeds with a small spoon. Be careful not to break the skins. Roughly chop the pulp and seeds and set them aside.
2. In a large pot of boiling salted water, cook the 4 hollowed-out zucchini for about 8 minutes or until tender. Carefully remove from the water and set aside.
3. Cut the remaining zucchini into quarters lengthwise and then into ¼-inch slices.
4. Preheat the oven to 350°.
5. In a medium-size sauté pan, combine the chopped pulp and seeds, zucchini slices, garlic, mushrooms, onion, and water. Cook over medium heat, uncovered, for about 35 minutes or until the water has evaporated. Remove from the heat and stir in the tarragon.
6. Stuff the zucchini shells with the vegetable mixture. Add salt and pepper to taste. Place the shells in a shallow baking dish and bake for about 15 minutes. Finish cooking them under the broiler for an additional 4 minutes or until the stuffing begins to brown.
7. Serve them on warm plates and garnish with the diced tomato and the chervil leaves.

Turnip Gratin with Onion and Thyme

<table>
<tr><td>

Serves 4

Carb Level: Moderate

Per serving:

Carbohydrate:	10.6 g
Protein:	3.5 g

Smaller turnips are generally more tender and flavorful in this recipe.

ॐ

</td></tr>
</table>

2 medium or 3 small turnips, peeled and cut into thin disks
1 small onion, peeled and sliced
1 teaspoon chopped fresh thyme
Salt and freshly ground black pepper to taste

1 pint heavy cream
2 tablespoons butter, plus extra for greasing
Chopped fresh parsley for garnish

1. Preheat oven to 350°.
2. Lightly butter a gratin dish. Place half of the turnip slices in the dish in an even layer. Layer all of the onion slices on top, sprinkle with the thyme and salt and pepper, and then with the rest of the turnip slices. Pour the cream over the top. Dot the top with butter, and bake for about 45 to 55 minutes, until the gratin is cooked through and brown and bubbly on top. To check for doneness, insert a thin-bladed knife into the center of the gratin. The blade should insert easily with minimal resistance. Allow to rest for at least 10 minutes before serving. Top with chopped parsley for added color.

 Vegetable Numbers

Carb counts for a ⅓-cup serving of the following vegetables:

Carrots	3.7 g
Eggplant	1.7 g
Spinach	0.7 g

CHAPTER 10

Lunch

Grilled Spicy Chicken Salad ❖	152
Hard-Boiled Egg Salad ❖	153
Pulled Chicken Salad ❖	153
Curried Chicken Chowder	154
Chicken Grape Salad ❖	155
Sautéed Sausage and Peppers ❖	156
Stuffed Tomato with Cottage Cheese ❖	157
Teriyaki Beef ❖	158
Spinach and Mushroom Rolls	159
Crab Cakes with Red Pepper Sauce	160
Broccoli Bacon Salad ❖	162
Vegetable Egg Salad ❖	162
Curried Chicken Spread ❖	163
Vegetable Cottage Cheese Spread ❖	163
Shrimp Salad ❖	164
Avocado with Tuna Salad ❖	164
New Orleans Muffuletta Salad ❖	165
Beef Roulade	166
Herb-Stuffed Flank Steak	168
Stuffed Cabbage Rolls	169
Layered Taco Salad ❖	170
Mushroom Curry Sauté ❖	171
Fresh Mozzarella Salad ❖	172
Beef Salad with Horseradish Dressing	173
Bacon, Lettuce, Tomato, and Cheese Salad ❖	174
Spinach Salad with Warm Bacon Dressing ❖	175
Hearts of Romaine with Parmesan Dressing ❖	176

❖ **Indicates Easy Recipe** ❖

Grilled Spicy Chicken Salad

Serves 4
Carb Level: Low

Per serving:	
Carbohydrate:	2.7 g
Protein:	39.0 g

Great with the Ranch Dressing (see page 109). Serve on a bed of crispy mixed greens.

∾

2 teaspoons seasoned salt
½ teaspoon each: garlic powder, onion powder, dried thyme, dried oregano, ground black pepper, paprika, and cayenne pepper

1½ pounds boneless, skinless chicken breasts
1 (15-ounce) package mixed baby greens

1. Mix all the seasoning ingredients in a small bowl to blend. Trim off any excess fat on the chicken breasts, rinse under cold running water, and pat dry with a paper towel. Dust each side of the chicken breasts with the seasoning.

2. Prepare a charcoal grill or preheat a gas grill to high. Make sure the grill grate is clean and lightly oiled to prevent sticking. Cook each side of the chicken for about 5 to 6 minutes, reducing heat or repositioning the chicken on the grill if too much charring is occurring. (Be careful not to overcook chicken, as the color from the spice mixture will bleed into the chicken.) Serve the warm chicken breasts over mixed baby greens with your choice of dressing.

Salt—There Is a Difference

Table salt is a fine-grained refined salt with additives that allow it to flow freely. Iodized salt is table salt with added iodine. Kosher salt is an additive-free coarse-grained salt. Sea salt is available in both fine-grain and coarse grain and is manufactured by evaporating sea water. Rock salt is somewhat gray in color and comes in large crystals. Pickling salt is an additive-free, fine-grain specifically used for brines.

Hard-Boiled Egg Salad

3 eggs, hard-boiled, peeled,
    cooled, and chopped
2 tablespoons minced celery
½ scallion, sliced
1 tablespoon chopped fresh dill
2 tablespoons mayonnaise

½ teaspoon Dijon mustard
Salt and freshly ground black
    pepper to taste

Mix all the ingredients together in a mixing bowl: stir just until combined. Adjust the salt and pepper to taste. Serve chilled.

Serves 2
Carb Level: Low

Per serving:	
Carbohydrate:	1.6 g
Protein:	10.6 g

You can add a little cayenne or Hungarian paprika to add some zip to this traditional recipe.

ϖ

Pulled Chicken Salad

1 small whole chicken, cooked
    rotisserie style
2 tablespoons scallion, minced
1 tablespoon parsley, chopped
3 tablespoons celery, diced fine
2 tablespoons capers, drained
    (or chopped stuffed olives)

1 tablespoon mayonnaise
1 tablespoon (or more) sour
    cream
Salt and freshly ground black
    pepper
2 whole lettuce leaves (optional)

When the chicken is cool enough to handle, pull the meat from the bones and cut it into medium-size pieces. Refrigerate the meat until completely cooled. Mix the minced scallion, parsley, celery, capers, mayonnaise, and sour cream until combined. Add the chicken and toss to coat evenly Add a pinch of salt and pepper, and adjust the amount of mayonnaise and sour cream to the desired consistency. Serve chilled over a lettuce leaf.

Serves 2
Carb Level: Low

Per serving (without added mayonnaise or sour cream):	
Carbohydrate:	1.4 g
Protein:	73.2 g

Most grocery stores carry rotisserie chickens hot and ready to take home. You can also substitute any leftover roast chicken meat.

ϖ

Curried Chicken Chowder

Serves 8

Carb Level: Moderate

Per serving:

Carbohydrate:	16.9 g
Protein:	21.7 g

This can be prepared 1 or 2 days ahead— reheat just before serving.

3-pound chicken, cut up into 8 pieces
3 cups thinly sliced carrots, divided
1 cup thinly sliced celery, with leaves
1 medium onion, quartered
4 whole cloves
1 tablespoon salt (optional)
1 bay leaf
10 cups water
3 tablespoons butter
8 ounces fresh mushrooms
1 tablespoon finely chopped shallot
½ teaspoon salt
½ teaspoon (or to taste) curry powder
¼ cup dry sherry
1 cup light cream
Avocado slices for garnish

1. Rinse the chicken under cold running water and pat dry with paper towels. Place the chicken pieces, 1 cup of the carrots, the celery, the onion quarters studded with the 4 cloves, the salt, and bay leaf in a 4-quart saucepan. Add enough water to cover, about 10 cups; bring to a boil, uncovered. Reduce to a simmer, partially cover, and cook on low for about 1 hour. Skim off and discard any residue that accumulates on the surface as it cooks.

2. Remove the chicken pieces and allow to cool. Pull the meat from the bones and discard the skin and bones. Cut the meat into ½-inch cubes; set aside.

3. Strain the chicken stock through a chinois or fine-mesh sieve. Reserve the stock and the vegetables; discard the cloves and the bay leaf. Let the stock sit for a few minutes, then skim off any fat that accumulates at the top.

4. Put the vegetables and 1 cup of stock into a food processor or blender. Blend until smooth in consistency. Heat the remaining stock in a large saucepan to boiling. Stir in the vegetable purée and the remaining carrots. Bring to a boil, then reduce heat to a simmer; cook, uncovered, for 30 minutes.

(recipe continues on the next page)

Curried Chicken Chowder (continued)

5. In a small skillet, heat the butter until it foams. Stir the mushrooms and shallot into the butter, and cook for 3 minutes. Stir in the salt and curry; cook over low heat for another 3 minutes. Stir the mushroom mixture into the chicken stock; simmer, uncovered, for 15 minutes.

6. Add the chicken pieces, sherry, and cream. Heat until hot and steaming, about 3 minutes, over medium heat—*do not boil*. Ladle into serving bowls and garnish with the avocado slices.

Chicken Grape Salad

2 cups cooked chicken breast,
   cut into small cubes
1 cup celery, chopped
1 cup seedless green or red
   grapes, halved
1 cup mayonnaise
1 tablespoon lemon juice
½ cup slivered almonds

½ teaspoon salt
Freshly ground black pepper
   to taste
Mixed greens

Combine all the ingredients except the mixed greens in a medium-size mixing bowl; toss well. Serve chilled over a bed of the mixed greens.

Serves 6
Carb Level: Low

Per serving:	
Carbohydrate:	5.2 g
Protein:	15.3 g

Serve with a glass of chilled chardonnay for a perfect pairing.

☙

Sautéed Sausage and Peppers

Serves 1

Carb Level: Low

Per serving:

Carbohydrate:	10.0 g
Protein:	18.2 g

It's easy to multiply this recipe for a small dinner for 2 to a group gathering.

2 tablespoons olive oil, divided
5 ounces Italian sausage
½ cup chopped zucchini
¼ cup chopped onion
½ cup trimmed, seeded, and chopped red bell pepper
Salt and freshly ground black pepper to taste

1. In a small sauté pan, heat 1 tablespoon of the olive oil on medium-high. Place the sausage in the pan: it should sizzle on contact. (If not, remove the sausage immediately and let the pan heat to the proper temperature.) Let the sausage caramelize to a medium golden brown color, turning as needed. Remove the sausage from the pan, set aside, and keep warm.
2. Add the remaining olive oil to the sauté pan, and add the zucchini, onion, and red pepper. Sauté, uncovered, stirring until the vegetable have softened and start to caramelize a bit; remove from heat. Sprinkle with salt and pepper, and toss.
3. To serve, cut the sausage links on a bias into thirds and place on a plate. Place the sautéed vegetables on top of the sausage. Serve immediately.

Where to Find Organic Foods

The Web site ✒ www.shopnatural.com is a good source for organic home and dry goods. The best organic produce is still purchased through your local Farmer's Market.

Stuffed Tomato with Cottage Cheese

⅓ cup cottage cheese
2 tablespoons minced fresh
   parsley
1 teaspoon minced garlic
Salt and freshly ground black
   pepper to taste

1 medium-size ripe tomato
1 tablespoon balsamic vinegar
½ cup mixed greens

Serves 1	
Carb Level: Low	
Per serving:	
Carbohydrate:	12.6 g
Protein:	12.6 g

Dice and add any left-over cheeses, deli meats, or veggies, or add fresh herbs and spices, to the cottage cheese mixture for a variation.

1. Mix together the cottage cheese, parsley, garlic, and salt and pepper (and anything else you would like); set aside.
2. Cut the very top off of the tomato. Scoop out the inside of the tomato with a melon baller or teaspoon. Discard the tomato top and inside pulp. Spoon the cottage cheese filling into the tomato.
3. On a serving dish, drizzle the vinegar over the mixed greens, and sprinkle with salt and pepper. Place the tomato over the top of the greens.

Fruit Facts

Note the following carb counts for a ½-cup serving of the following fresh fruits: fresh mango, 14.0 grams; fresh pineapple, 9.6 grams; fresh apples, 8.4 grams; fresh raspberries, 7.1 grams; fresh blueberries, 10.2 grams; fresh strawberries, 5.2 grams; fresh pears, 12.5 grams; fresh red grapes, 13.9 grams; fresh green grapes, 13.7 grams.

Teriyaki Beef

Serves 6
Carb Level: Low

Per serving:	
Carbohydrate:	9.1 g
Protein:	24.3 g

These skewers also make great appetizers. Prepare them the evening before if you like, then grill or broil just before serving.

∾

Marinade:

¼ cup rice wine vinegar
½ cup teriyaki sauce
¼ cup canola oil
1 tablespoon dry white sherry
1 small clove garlic, minced
1 (1-inch) piece fresh ginger, crushed

1½ pounds boneless beef sirloin, cut into ⅛-inch slices
Wooden skewers, soaked in water
6 cups julienned Boston lettuce
¼ cup of your favorite vinaigrette (see vinaigrette recipes in Chapter 7)
½ cup chopped red onion

1. Combine all the marinade ingredients in a shallow casserole dish; mix to combine. Add the beef to the dish and thoroughly coat all the pieces with the marinade. Cover and refrigerate for 1 to 2 hours or overnight.
2. Prepare a charcoal grill or preheat a gas grill to high. Make sure the grill grate is clean and lightly oiled to prevent sticking.
3. Thread the marinated meat onto wooden skewers that have been soaked in water. Cook the skewers for 1 or 2 minutes on each side until the desired temperature is achieved.
4. Serve the hot skewers on a bed of the Boston lettuce topped with the vinaigrette and garnished with the red onion.

Spinach and Mushroom Rolls

1 (10-ounce) package frozen
    chopped spinach, thawed,
    water squeezed out, and
    cooked according to
    package directions
4 eggs, separated
Salt and freshly ground black
    pepper to taste
1/4 cup grated Parmesan
    cheese

Filling:

1 tablespoon butter
2 cups sliced medium-size
    mushrooms
1 tablespoon all-purpose flour
2/3 cup milk
Pinch of nutmeg
Salt and freshly ground black
    pepper to taste

Serves 4	
Carb Level: Low	
Per serving:	
Carbohydrate:	8.5 g
Protein:	14.6 g

You can top the rolls with the Tomato Sauce on page 67.

✎

1. Preheat oven to 400°. Line a jellyroll pan with nonstick parchment paper and then oil lightly.
2. Drain the spinach well and place it in a large bowl. Beat the 4 egg yolks well then thoroughly mix them into the chopped spinach. Season to taste with salt and pepper.
3. Whisk the 4 egg whites in a large grease-free bowl until just holding their shape (soft peaks). Using a metal spoon, quickly fold them into the spinach mixture. Spoon the mixture into the prepared jellyroll pan, spreading it across entire pan. Sprinkle the grated Parmesan cheese over the entire surface; bake for 10 minutes.
4. Meanwhile, make the filling: Heat the butter in a small saucepan. Add the sliced mushrooms and cook gently until softened. Stir in the flour; cook, stirring constantly, for 1 minute. Slowly stir in the milk, and cook the sauce until thickened. Stir in the nutmeg and season to taste.
5. Remove the spinach roulade from the oven and invert onto a sheet of waxed paper. Quickly spread the mushroom filling over the surface and gently roll up the roulade. Cut into thick slices and serve immediately. Gently reheat the rolls in the oven as necessary.

Crab Cakes with Red Pepper Sauce

Serves 6
Carb Level: Low

Per serving:

Carbohydrate:	9.3 g
Protein:	18.3 g

Cooked crab cakes freeze well for up to 3 weeks. Thaw overnight in the refrigerator and reheat at 375° in the oven until crispy hot.

Crab Cakes:

¼ teaspoon salt
1½ tablespoons paprika
1½ tablespoons fresh ground black pepper
1 teaspoon (or to taste) onion powder
½ teaspoon cayenne pepper
1 teaspoon fresh thyme leaves
¼ teaspoon dried oregano
½ teaspoon white pepper
1½ tablespoons minced garlic
⅓ cup bread crumbs
1½ tablespoons Romano or Parmesan cheese
1 tablespoon minced fresh parsley
1 pound fresh or frozen crabmeat, picked over for shells
½ cup mayonnaise
2 tablespoons chopped scallions, white part only
3 tablespoons chopped green bell pepper
4 tablespoons diced onion
2 tablespoons chopped celery
⅛ teaspoon Tabasco sauce
1 teaspoon Worcestershire sauce
½ cup corn oil

Red Pepper Sauce:

1 red bell pepper, roasted in the oven
   until cooked, seeded
1 clove garlic, minced
½ cup mayonnaise
¼ cup sour cream
Salt and freshly ground black pepper to taste

(recipe continues on the next page)

Crab Cakes with Red Pepper Sauce (continued)

1. To prepare the crab cakes: Mix together the salt, paprika, black pepper, onion powder, cayenne, thyme, oregano, and white pepper, then add the minced garlic; set aside.

2. Mix together the bread crumbs, Romano cheese, and parsley; set aside.

3. In a bowl, blend $1\frac{1}{2}$ teaspoons of the seasoning mix with all of the remaining crab cake ingredients *except* the corn oil and the bread crumb mixture. Form into $1\frac{1}{2}$-inch balls. Roll them in the breadcrumb mixture and flatten into $\frac{1}{2}$-inch-thick patties.

4. Heat half of the corn oil in a skillet over medium heat. Sauté the crab cakes in batches until golden brown on each side. Replenish the corn oil as needed. Transfer the cakes to paper towels after cooked to drain; keep warm.

5. To prepare the sauce: In a food processor or blender, combine all of the ingredients; process until smooth. Serve the crab cakes with the red pepper sauce on the side.

Broccoli Bacon Salad

Serves 12
Carb Level: Low

Per serving:

Carbohydrate:	4.6 g
Protein:	5.6 g

You can substitute frozen chopped broccoli, cooked according to package directions, if you are in a time pinch.

2 bunches broccoli, chopped, cooked crisp-tender, drained
8 bacon strips, cooked and crumbled
1½ cups shredded Cheddar cheese
1 medium-size red onion, chopped
¼ cup red wine vinegar
2 tablespoons honey
¾ cup mayonnaise
1 tablespoon fresh lemon juice
1 teaspoon salt
½ teaspoon freshly ground black pepper

In a large bowl, combine the cooled broccoli, bacon, cheese, and onion. Prepare the dressing by whisking together all the remaining ingredients. Pour the dressing over the broccoli mixture and toss to combine. Cover and refrigerate until ready to use.

Vegetable Egg Salad

Serves 4
Carb Level: Low

Per serving:

Carbohydrate:	4.5 g
Protein:	8.7 g

Goes great on a bed of fresh greens. This salad holds up well refrigerated for 1 or 2 days.

4 hard-boiled eggs, peeled and chopped
2 ounces medium-firm tofu, drained and diced
½ cup thinly sliced celery
¼ cup chopped onion
1 tablespoon chopped fresh parsley
1 tablespoon chopped fresh dill
Salt and freshly ground black pepper to taste
1 teaspoon Worcestershire sauce
4 tablespoons mayonnaise
½ cup frozen green peas, thawed and drained

Combine all the ingredients *except* the peas in a medium-size bowl; mix well. Add the peas and toss gently. Cover and chill before serving.

Curried Chicken Spread

1 pound boneless, skinless
   chicken breasts, cooked and
   cut into medium-size dice
2/3 cup sour cream
1/2 cup chopped pineapple
   (fresh or canned)

1/2 teaspoon curry powder
1/2 cup chopped celery
Salt and freshly ground black
   pepper to taste

Place the chicken in the work bowl of a food process. Pulse until the cooked chicken meat resembles the consistency of canned tuna. In a bowl, mix together the chicken and the remaining ingredients.

Serves 2
Carb Level: Low

Per serving:	
Carbohydrate:	9.5 g
Protein:	44.8 g

Great as a spread on vegetables or rolled up in lettuce leaves.

Vegetable Cottage Cheese Spread

1 (12-ounce) container cottage
   cheese
1 teaspoon dried whole savory
1/2 cup seeded and diced
   tomato
1/3 cup shredded carrot
1/3 cup unpeeled chopped
   cucumber

1/3 cup chopped green bell
   pepper
1/4 cup sliced green onions
1 tablespoon red wine vinegar
Salt and freshly ground black
   pepper to taste

Combine the cottage cheese and savory, stirring well. Add the remaining ingredients; toss gently. Serve chilled on a bed of lettuce greens.

Serves 4
Carb Level: Low

Per serving:	
Carbohydrate:	6.3 g
Protein:	12.1 g

Add a variety of different fresh chopped herbs for a different flavor.

Shrimp Salad

Serves 6
Carb Level: Low

Per serving:

Carbohydrate:	3.1 g
Protein:	17.0 g

Simple and satisfying. Serve on a bed of baby spinach leaves with a light vinaigrette dressing.

1 pound small shrimp, peeled and cooked
1 hard-boiled egg, chopped
1½ tablespoons chopped celery
1½ tablespoons chopped dill pickle
2 tablespoons thinly sliced shallot
2 tablespoons chopped yellow onion
2 tablespoons mayonnaise
1 teaspoon Dijon mustard
Salt and freshly ground black pepper to taste
1 tablespoon paprika

Combine the shrimp, egg, celery, pickle, shallot, and onion in a large bowl. Mix the mayonnaise and mustard together in a small bowl. Add the mayonnaise mixture to the shrimp and toss to coat. Salt and pepper to taste, and garnish with paprika.

Avocado with Tuna Salad

Serves 1
Carb Level: Moderate

Per serving:

Carbohydrate:	13.1 g
Protein:	27.6 g

A great entrée salad luncheon dish. You can also serve the tuna salad in Boston lettuce leaf wraps.

3 ounces albacore tuna, flaked
2 tablespoons mayonnaise
1 teaspoon Dijon mustard
1 hard-boiled egg, chopped
½ scallion, minced
1 teaspoon chopped fresh dill
Salt and freshly ground black pepper to taste
¼ cup extra-virgin olive oil
2 tablespoons red wine vinegar
½ cup mixed greens
½ avocado
3 black olives, quartered, for garnish
1 pickle, sliced, for garnish

In a mixing bowl, mix together the tuna, mayonnaise, Dijon, egg, scallion, dill, and salt and pepper. In another small bowl, whisk together the olive oil and vinegar; season with salt and pepper. Toss the mixed greens with the vinaigrette; place on plate. Slice the avocado and fan it across the dressed greens. Top with the tuna salad. Garnish with the black olives and pickle.

New Orleans Muffuletta Salad

½ cup chopped fresh broccoli florets

½ cup chopped fresh cauliflower florets

¼ cup finely chopped celery

1 cup finely chopped pimento-stuffed olives, with ¼ cup liquid from the jar

4 cloves garlic, finely chopped

¼ cup extra-virgin olive oil

¼ teaspoon freshly ground black pepper

4 cups chopped iceberg lettuce, rinsed and patted dry

¼ pound Genoa salami, thinly sliced

¼ pound prosciutto, thinly sliced

¼ pound provolone, thinly sliced and cut into quarters

½ cup vinaigrette salad dressing

Serves 4	
Carb Level: Low	
Per serving:	
Carbohydrate:	10.0 g
Protein:	21.7 g

Makes a great luncheon entrée salad—a simple stop at the deli counter and produce counter is all you need.

1. In a medium-size bowl, combine the broccoli, cauliflower, celery, olives, olive juice, garlic, olive oil, and black pepper. Let this mixture, called gardiniere, stand for at least 1 hour.
2. Place the lettuce in a bowl or on a platter. Top the lettuce with the salami, prosciutto, and provolone, then spoon some of the gardiniere on top. Serve with your favorite vinaigrette.

More Fruit Please!

How many carbs are in a ½-cup serving of the following fresh fruits? Fresh cherries, 12.4 grams; fresh kiwi fruit, 15.1 grams; fresh cantaloupe, 6.7 grams; fresh honeydew melon, 7.8 grams; fresh watermelon, 5.7 grams; fresh bananas, 26.2 grams.

Beef Roulade

Serves 4
Carb Level: Moderate

Per serving:

Carbohydrate:	18.2 g
Protein:	64.3 g

You can prepare this in advance and gently reheat before serving. Just be careful not to let the beef dry out or overcook.

Brown Sauce:

4 tablespoons vegetable oil
½ peeled carrot, sliced
½ stalk celery, chopped
½ yellow onion, chopped
1 clove garlic, chopped
4 tablespoons all-purpose flour
1 quart beef stock
1 bay leaf
2 peppercorns
¼ cup tomato purée
⅛ cup chopped tomatoes

Beef roulade:

2 strips bacon, diced
½ pound ground beef
½ cup chopped yellow onion
1 clove garlic, chopped
2 eggs
3 tablespoons brown mustard
¼ cup milk
1½ cups bread crumbs
1 tablespoon chopped fresh parsley
1 teaspoon salt
1 teaspoon freshly ground black pepper
4 thinly sliced rounds of beef
4 thin strips sour pickle
2 tablespoons butter
Chopped fresh parsley for garnish

(recipe continues on the next page)

Beef Roulade (continued)

1. To prepare the brown sauce: Heat the oil in a large sauce pot or Dutch oven over medium-high heat. Add the carrot, celery, onion, and garlic; braise until light brown. Add the flour and stir well; cook until the flour turns brown, stirring so that it browns evenly. Add the remaining sauce ingredients; bring to a boil, reduce heat, and let simmer slowly for 1 hour, stirring occasionally. Strain into a bowl; discard solids.

2. Preheat oven to 325°.

3. In a medium-size sauté pan, sauté the bacon, ground beef, onion, and garlic until lightly browned; let cool. Transfer the sautéed mixture to a large mixing bowl and add the eggs, mustard, milk, bread crumbs, parsley, salt, and pepper; mix well.

4. Spread the mixture equally on the slices of beef. Place a pickle strip on top of the mixture and then roll up each beef slice; secure closed with toothpicks or tie with a string. Melt the butter in a sauté pan over medium heat and brown the roulades on all sides. Place the roulades in a baking pan and cover with the hot brown sauce; bake until tender, approximately $1\frac{1}{2}$ to 2 hours. Sprinkle with a little chopped parsley and serve.

The Importance of Soy Sauce

Soy sauce is a key flavoring agent in Asian cooking. It is manufactured by fermenting boiled soy beans and roasted wheat or barley. It should be used sparingly in recipes due to its intense salty flavor and carbohydrate count. Soy sauce contains 6.1 grams of carbohydrates per $\frac{1}{4}$ cup.

Herb-Stuffed Flank Steak

Serves 4

Carb Level: Moderate

Per serving:

Carbohydrate:	14.8 g
Protein:	37.4 g

Make sure to cook the stuffed meat completely through, as there is raw egg in the filling.

2 pounds beef flank steak
2 tablespoons butter
½ large onion, chopped
3 cloves garlic, crushed
½ cup sliced mushrooms
¼ cup chopped fresh parsley
½ cup soft bread crumbs
½ teaspoon dried basil leaves
½ teaspoon dried oregano leaves

Salt and freshly ground black pepper to taste
4 ounces cream cheese
1 egg, slightly beaten
2 tablespoons olive oil
1 cup dry red wine

1. Preheat oven to 350°.
2. Pound the steak on both sides with a meat mallet to flatten evenly to about ⅛-inch thickness. In medium-size sauté pan, heat the butter over medium-high heat. When the butter is foaming, add the onion and sauté for about 3 minutes. Add the garlic and sauté for 1 more minute. Add the mushrooms and cook until soft, about 3 minutes. Add the parsley, bread crumbs, basil, oregano, salt and pepper, cream cheese, and egg; mix well.
3. Spread the mixture on the steak. Roll lengthwise, jellyroll style, and tie with string approximately every 2 inches. In a large skillet over high heat, brown the meat on all sides in the olive oil. Transfer to a baking dish. Add the wine, cover, and bake for 2 hours. Cut into 1-inch-thick slices and serve with the pan juices.

Stuffed Cabbage Rolls

1 head cabbage
3 pounds lean ground beef
2 teaspoons salt
1/4 teaspoon fresh ground
   black pepper
1 small onion, minced
1 (8-ounce) can tomato sauce

Sauce:

1/3 cup whipping cream
1 tablespoon honey
1/4 cup vinegar
1 (8-ounce) can tomato sauce
1/4 cup chopped parsley

Serves 6
Carb Level: Moderate

Per serving:	
Carbohydrate:	16.8 g
Protein:	41.5 g

Great made in quantity for a casual afternoon lunch.

∾

1. Remove the core from the cabbage head, keeping the head whole. Bring a large pot of salted water to a boil and drop the cabbage in for 4 to 6 minutes. (This will make it easier to separate and remove the leaves.) Pull off 12 whole leaves from the cabbage head.

2. In a medium-size bowl, combine the beef, salt, pepper, onion, and tomato sauce; blend well. Place the cabbage leaves in a very large bowl. Bring a large pot of water to a boil, then immediately cover the cabbage with the boiled water. Let stand for 5 minutes. Drain well.

3. Shape the meat mixture into 12 miniature loaf shapes. Place 1 loaf in the center of each cabbage leaf; roll up, folding in the sides. Place the rolls, seam side down, in a 10-inch sauté pan or skillet.

4. Combine all the sauce ingredients. Pour the sauce evenly over the cabbage rolls; bring to a boil, reduce heat to a simmer, and cover. Cook, basting often, for about 1 to 1½ hours.

Layered Taco Salad

Serves 4
Carb Level: Moderate

Per serving:	
Carbohydrate:	18.1 g
Protein:	20.0 g

Add cooked chicken or ground beef to make this an even better tasting entrée luncheon salad.

∽

½ cup mayonnaise
1 cup sour cream
½ teaspoon chili powder
½ teaspoon onion powder
½ teaspoon cumin
½ teaspoon garlic powder
1 teaspoon salt
1 teaspoon black pepper
¼ teaspoon red pepper flakes
4 cups shredded lettuce

8 ounces Cheddar cheese, shredded
8 ounces Swiss cheese, shredded
2 ripe tomatoes, finely chopped
1 (3½-ounce) can chopped ripe black olives
½ small bunch green onions, finely chopped

In a medium-size mixing bowl, combine the mayonnaise, sour cream, chili powder, onion powder, cumin, garlic powder, salt, pepper, and red pepper flakes; whisk together until well blended. Spread evenly on a serving platter with sides. Top with the shredded lettuce, then the cheeses, then the tomatoes, black olives, and lastly, the green onions. Cover and refrigerate overnight. Serve with a little salsa on the side.

Mushroom Curry Sauté

2 onions, chopped
½ stick of butter
1 teaspoon tomato paste
1 teaspoon ground cinnamon
½ teaspoon garam masala or
    curry powder
½ teaspoon ground cloves
4 cups sliced medium-size
    mushrooms
3–4 dashes dry white wine
    (water can be substituted)

⅔ cup sour cream
1 cup chicken stock
¼ teaspoon chili powder
Salt and freshly ground black
    pepper to taste
Fresh cilantro leaves for
    garnish

Serves 4
Carb Level: Moderate

Per serving:	
Carbohydrate:	12.6 g
Protein:	4.0 g

This is a great way to dress up domestic button mushrooms. Premade garam masala is available in the spice section of most supermarkets.

1. In a large sauté pan over medium-high heat, sauté the onions in the butter until golden brown. Add the tomato paste, cinnamon, garam masala (*or* curry), and ground cloves; cook, stirring constantly, for 4 to 5 minutes.

2. Add the mushrooms and a few drops of white wine. Cook, stirring constantly, for 4 to 5 minutes. Gradually add the sour cream, and cook for another 3 to 5 minutes. Add the stock and simmer for 15 minutes. Add the chili powder and salt and pepper. Garnish with fresh cilantro leaves. Can be served hot or room temperature.

Fresh Mozzarella Salad

Serves 2
Carb Level: Moderate

Per serving:	
Carbohydrate:	15.3 g
Protein:	46.4 g

You can always substitute the traditional tomato for the roasted peppers.

❧

4 large red bell peppers
2 balls fresh mozzarella cheese
  (about ¾ pound total)
16 large basil leaves

Extra-virgin olive oil
Salt and freshly ground black
  pepper to taste

1. Roast the peppers directly on the range over high heat, turning them until they are evenly blackened. Place the peppers in a medium-size bowl and cover with plastic wrap. (This allows them to steam, making it easier to peel them.) Once they are cool enough to handle, rinse them under cold running water and peel off the skins (the skin should come off very easily). Cut off the stems, then slice away the ribs and remove the seeds. Quarter the peppers by slicing them lengthwise.

2. Slice the mozzarella balls into ¼-inch-thick rounds and arrange the slices on a serving platter, alternating them with the pepper quarters. Place the basil leaves in between the mozzarella and peppers. Drizzle with extra-virgin olive oil and sprinkle with salt and pepper, then serve.

Beef Salad
with Horseradish Dressing

½ pound green beans
1½ cups packaged, peeled
   baby carrots
12 ounces beef sirloin steak,
   cut 1-inch thick
Salt and freshly ground black
   pepper to taste

4 cups mixed salad greens
1 cup Creamy Horseradish
   Dressing (see recipe on
   page 110)

Serves 4
Carb Level: Moderate

Per serving:

Carbohydrate:	18.6 g
Protein:	20.6 g

Try it with Ranch Dressing (see page 109) for a variation.

ॐ

1. Wash the green beans and trim off the ends. Cut the beans in half crosswise. In a covered medium-size saucepan, cook the beans in boiling salted water until tender and a vibrant green. Add the baby carrots and cook for another 10 to 15 minutes or until the vegetables are tender. Drain and rinse under cold running water. Cover and chill for 4 to 24 hours.

2. Trim the fat from the meat. Sprinkle both sides with salt and pepper. Place the meat on the unheated rack of a broiler pan; broil 3 to 4 inches from the heat to desired doneness, turning once. Allow 10 to 12 minutes per inch of thickness for medium-rare or 12 to 15 minutes for medium. Let rest, tented with tin foil, for 5 minutes after cooking. Thinly slice across the grain into bite-size strips.

3. Divide the greens among individual plates or on 1 large plate. Arrange the green beans, baby carrots, and meat slices on top of the salad greens. Spoon the Creamy Horseradish Dressing over the top.

Bacon, Lettuce, Tomato, and Cheese Salad

Serves 2
Carb Level: Moderate

Per serving:	
Carbohydrate:	19.5 g
Protein:	27.1 g

Everyone's favorite sandwich, without the bread—this is a satisfying lunch treat.

～

10 smoked bacon slices
$1/4$ teaspoon minced garlic
1 tablespoon fresh-squeezed
   lemon juice
$1/4$ cup mayonnaise
1 tablespoon snipped chives
1 tablespoon water
Salt and pepper to taste

1 small red onion, thinly sliced
$1/2$ pound cherry tomatoes,
   halved
1 cup shredded Monterey jack
   cheese
1 head Romaine lettuce, torn
   into bite-size pieces

In a skillet, cook the bacon over medium heat until crisp. Drain the bacon on paper towels, then crumble. In a small bowl, whisk together the garlic, lemon juice, mayonnaise, chives, water, and salt and pepper. In a large bowl toss together the onion, tomatoes, cheese, lettuce, half of the bacon, and enough of the prepared dressing to coat. Serve the salad on a platter and top with the remaining bacon.

Variations on an Old Favorite

BLTs can still be a favorite. Use Farmer's Market ripe tomatoes, scoop out the seeds and inner membrane and fill with a mixture of crispy chopped bacon, fine diced tomatoes, and chopped lettuce lightly dressed with mayonnaise. Top with blue cheese crumbles if desired and serve on a bed of crispy greens—you'll never miss the bread. One medium whole tomato contains about 5 grams of carbohydrates and is loaded with vitamin C as well as potassium and other minerals.

Spinach Salad
with Warm Bacon Dressing

*1 pound tender young spinach,
  trimmed of coarse stems*
*6 slices bacon, chopped cross-
  wise into julienne strips*
*4 green onions, washed,
  trimmed, and thinly sliced*
*1 clove garlic, peeled and
  crushed*
1 tablespoon ketchup

½ cup red wine vinegar
½ teaspoon salt
¼ teaspoon black pepper

Serves 4
Carb Level: Moderate

Per serving:	
Carbohydrate:	18.2 g
Protein:	9.0 g

You can make this dressing ahead of time and refrigerate it—reheat it in the microware, then dress the salad.

∾

1. Wash the spinach well in several changes of cold water, dry very well, then bundle in paper towels and refrigerate while preparing dressing.
2. To prepare the dressing, brown the bacon in a large heavy skillet over medium heat for 3 to 5 minutes, until crisp. Remove the bacon with a slotted spoon and set it aside on paper towels to drain.
3. Add the green onions and garlic to the bacon drippings in the pan and sauté over low heat for about 2 minutes, until soft. Mix in the remaining ingredients and bring to a boil. Mound the spinach in a large heat-proof salad bowl. Pour the mixture over the spinach, sprinkle in the bacon bits, and toss well to mix. Serve immediately.

Hearts of Romaine
with Parmesan Dressing

1 heart of romaine, outer leaves removed

2 teaspoons white wine vinegar

2 tablespoons extra-virgin olive oil

⅔ cup freshly grated Parmesan cheese

Salt and freshly ground black pepper to taste

Separate the romaine leaves. In a large bowl, whisk together the vinegar, oil, half of the Parmesan, and salt and pepper. Toss the romaine leaves with the dressing and serve sprinkled with the remaining Parmesan.

CHAPTER 11

Comfort Food

Deviled Eggs ❖	178
Lime-Broiled Catfish ❖	179
Salmon with Chive Mustard Butter	180
Baby Back Ribs with Sauerkraut	181
Fried Chicken	182
Crustless Salmon Potpie	183
Spicy Chicken Wings ❖	184
Baked Pork Chops with Caramelized Onions and Smoked Cheddar	185
Stuffed Bell Peppers	186
Pot Roast with Vegetable Sauce	187
Classic Meat Loaf	188
Chicken Potpie Stew	189

❖ Indicates Easy Recipe ❖

Deviled Eggs

Serves 2

Carb Level: Low

Per serving:

Carbohydrate:	1.6 g
Protein:	13.0 g

Everyone's favorite—a great addition to salads or as a whole foods protein supplement.

4 large eggs
2½ tablespoons mayonnaise
1½ teaspoons Dijon mustard
Hot red pepper sauce to taste

Salt and freshly ground white pepper to taste
2 tablespoons minced fresh chives

1. Place the eggs in a medium-size saucepan and cover with water. Bring to a boil, reduce to a simmer, and cook for 9 minutes. Plunge the eggs into a bowl filled with ice water. Allow the eggs to cool completely.
2. Carefully peel the shells from the eggs. Cut the eggs in half and remove the yolks from the whites. Place the yolks in a bowl and add the mayonnaise, mustard, hot pepper sauce, salt and pepper, and chives. With the back of a fork, mash all of the ingredients until blended.
3. Fill the egg whites with the yolk mixture using a teaspoon or a pastry bag fitted with a star tip. Serve chilled.

Lime-Broiled Catfish

2 tablespoons butter
2 tablespoons fresh-squeezed
    lime juice
1 teaspoon finely grated lime
    zest
¼ teaspoon garlic powder
¼ teaspoon paprika

Salt and freshly ground black
    pepper to taste
2 (6-ounce) catfish fillets,
    boned, skin on

Serves 2
Carb Level: Low

Per serving:	
Carbohydrate:	1.8 g
Protein:	26.3 g

A favorite recipe from
the South.

∾

1. Melt the butter in a medium-size sauté pan over medium-low heat.
   Stir in the lime juice, lime zest, garlic powder, paprika, and salt and
   pepper to taste; set aside.
2. Preheat the broiler.
3. Season the catfish fillets with salt and pepper. Brush each fillet generously with the lime sauce. Place the fish, skin side down, on an oiled
   baking sheet and broil for about 6 to 8 minutes or until done. Add
   any leftover lime marinade to the pan juices, heat, and spoon over the
   fillets. Serve immediately.

Salmon
with Chive Mustard Butter

Serves 6
Carb Level: Low

Per serving:	
Carbohydrate:	1.2 g
Protein:	12.3 g

Sea bass or snapper can be substituted for the salmon.

1½ tablespoons stone-ground Dijon mustard

1½ teaspoons finely grated orange zest

3½ tablespoons fresh-squeezed lemon juice, divided

¾ teaspoon salt

¼ teaspoon freshly ground black pepper

8 tablespoons unsalted butter, softened

5 tablespoons finely chopped fresh chives, divided

3 pounds salmon fillets, boned and skin on

1. In a medium-size bowl, combine the mustard, orange zest, 1½ tablespoons lemon juice, salt, pepper, butter, and 3 tablespoons of chives; mix well to blend.
2. Preheat oven to 425°.
3. In a lightly buttered baking dish, place the fillets skin side down. Brush each fillet with the remaining lemon juice and season with salt and pepper. Spread about 2 to 2½ tablespoons of the butter mixture over each fillet to coat evenly.
4. Bake for about 12 minutes or until done. To check for doneness, insert a thin-bladed knife into the thickest part of the fillet. The flesh should flake and separate easily and there should be no trace of translucence. The fish should be opaque and flaky. Transfer the fish to a warm platter and brush any remaining mustard chive butter over the fish while it is hot. Sprinkle with the remaining chives to garnish. Cut each fillet in half to serve.

Cooking Times for Fish

As a rule of thumb, you can expect fish to take about 12 minutes per inch to cook through in a preheated 425° oven.

Baby Back Ribs with Sauerkraut

1 (32-ounce) container sauerkraut, drained and rinsed
3 cups shredded red cabbage
2 tablespoons, plus 1 teaspoon
  paprika
4 cloves garlic, minced

1 (14½-ounce) can stewed
  tomatoes
3 pounds pork baby back ribs,
  trimmed of fat
Salt and freshly ground black
  pepper to taste

Serves 4
Carb Level: Moderate

Per serving:	
Carbohydrate:	19.5 g
Protein:	37.2 g

Definitely a home-style entrée. This is a great dish for a casual family get-together.

∾

1. In a medium-size bowl, combine the sauerkraut, cabbage, 1 teaspoon of paprika, garlic, and tomatoes; stir well to mix. Spread this mixture into the bottom of a large oiled baking dish.
2. Preheat oven to 375°.
3. Arrange the ribs on top of the sauerkraut mixture, curved side up. Season with salt and pepper and the rest of the paprika. Bake in the oven, covered with foil, for about 1½ hours or until the meat is tender. Uncover the pan, turn the ribs over, and bake for another 20 minutes (uncovered).
4. To serve, cut the ribs apart from the bones and serve over the sauerkraut.

Sauerkraut

Always thought of as a German creation, sauerkraut was eaten by Chinese laborers of the Great Wall of China over 2,000 years ago. Chinese sauerkraut was made from shredded cabbage and fermented in rice wine. Eventually it found its way to Europe where it has become a food staple. Quality sauerkraut can be purchased in jars or cans at the supermarket. Fresh kraut is available in delicatessens and in plastic bags in the refrigerated foods section of supermarkets. All krauts should be rinsed before being used. Sauerkraut is an excellent source of vitamin C and some B vitamins. A ⅓-cup serving contains 3.4 grams of carbohydrates.

Fried Chicken

1½ cups buttermilk
3-pound whole chicken, cut into 8 serving pieces
½ cup all-purpose flour
1½ teaspoons salt
½ teaspoon black pepper
1 teaspoon paprika
½ teaspoon garlic powder
Large pinch of grated nutmeg
Oil for deep-frying
Fresh parsley sprigs for garnish

1. Pour the buttermilk into a large nonmetallic bowl. Add the chicken pieces to the buttermilk and turn to coat. Cover and refrigerate, turning occasionally, for 2 to 3 hours.
2. In a large bowl, combine the flour with the salt, pepper, paprika, garlic powder, and nutmeg. Remove the chicken pieces from the buttermilk and shake off any excess liquid. Allow to drain. Toss the chicken pieces in a large plastic food storage bag with the flour mixture to ensure the pieces are evenly coated.
3. Pour ¾ inch of oil into a deep skillet and heat to 350°. Use a deep-fry thermometer to get an accurate reading.
4. Fry the chicken in batches to avoid overcrowding the pan. Cook for about 10 to 15 minutes, turning occasionally so the pieces cook to an even crispy golden brown. Drain the chicken on paper towels. Transfer to a large platter and garnish with fresh parsley sprigs.

Jell-O?

Jell-O is known as one of the old-fashioned favorites for comfort foods. Jell-O has become modernized with its sugar-free version, which is great for low-carb desserts.

Crustless Salmon Potpie

2 pounds salmon fillets
5 tablespoons canola oil,
   divided
Salt and freshly ground black
   pepper to taste
1¾ cups cleaned and thinly
   sliced leeks, white parts only
1½ cups thinly sliced fennel
   bulbs
5 tablespoons butter

5 tablespoons all-purpose flour
2½ cups milk
6 tablespoons fresh-squeezed
   lemon juice
Salt and freshly ground black
   pepper to taste
2 tablespoons chopped fresh
   dill for garnish

Serves 8
Carb Level: Moderate

Per serving:	
Carbohydrate:	10.2 g
Protein:	21.1 g

A great hearty winter dish. Use quality center-cut fillets for the best results.

∾

1. Preheat the oven to 425°.
2. Brush the salmon fillets with 1 tablespoon of oil and season with salt and pepper. Lightly oil a baking sheet. Bake for about 8 to 12 minutes or until the centers are just cooked. Remove from the pan and let cool. Remove the skin and cut into 1-inch pieces. (The salmon may flake apart.)
3. Heat the remaining oil in a large sauté pan over medium heat. Add the leeks and fennel, and cook for about 5 minutes or until tender. Remove from the heat and add to the salmon pieces.
4. Melt the butter in a medium-size saucepan over medium heat. Add the flour and cook, stirring, until well blended. Gradually pour in the milk, whisking constantly until slightly thickened. Add the lemon juice a little at a time according to taste. Season with salt and pepper. Add the salmon and vegetables and heat to just bubbling. Serve in warm bowls and garnish with chopped dill.

Where to Buy Fresh Fish

If you don't have a reliable fresh fish provider, try a reputable local sushi restaurant. They may be willing to sell you a piece of salmon. Use the freshest, highest quality fish you can find.

Spicy Chicken Wings

Serves 10

Carb Level: Moderate

Per serving:

Carbohydrate:	18.2 g
Protein:	10.9 g

Serve with blue cheese dressing and celery ribs to complete this homey appetizer dish.

1 cup white wine vinegar
2 tablespoons red pepper sauce, preferably Tabasco
2 tablespoons honey
2 tablespoons soy sauce
2 tablespoons dried thyme leaves
2 tablespoons cayenne pepper
4 tablespoons garlic powder

4 teaspoons salt
2 pounds chicken wings, split at joints into 2 pieces, wing tips removed
1 bunch green onions, cleaned and chopped

1. Combine the vinegar, pepper sauce, honey, soy sauce, thyme, cayenne, garlic powder, and salt in a large resealable plastic bag. Add the chicken wings and toss well to coat. Refrigerate overnight.
2. Preheat oven to 375°.
3. Line a baking sheet with foil and brush it lightly with oil. Drain the chicken, reserving the marinade. Arrange the chicken on the baking sheet. Place the marinade in a medium-size saucepan over medium-high heat and cook for about 6 minutes or until reduced by half. Brush the wings generously on all sides with the reduced marinade.
4. Bake the wings for about 30 minutes. Turn the wings and bake for 15 more minutes. Serve on a platter garnished with the chopped green onion.

Remember Grandma's Latkes

You can still enjoy the same satisfying taste and flavor of Grandma's latkes by substituting low carbohydrate zucchini for the potatoes. Prepare in the same method as potato latkes but keep the pancakes a little smaller for quicker cooking.

Baked Pork Chops with Caramelized Onions and Smoked Cheddar

8 (7- to 8-ounce) lean center-cut
    pork chops (¾- to 1-inch
    thick), trimmed of excess fat
Salt and freshly ground black
    pepper to taste
4 tablespoons canola oil, plus
    more if needed
8 cups sliced onions
1 teaspoon sugar
4 teaspoons chopped garlic
4-5 cups beef broth
¾- cup grated smoked
    Cheddar (3 ounces grated
    with the rind)
3 tablespoons chopped fresh
    flat-leaf parsley for garnish

Serves 8	
Carb Level: Moderate	
Per serving:	
Carbohydrate:	16.9 g
Protein:	39.7 g

A great do-ahead.
The flavor improves
when allowed to sit
refrigerated overnight;
then gently reheat just
before serving.

1. Preheat oven to 350°.
2. Season both sides of the pork chops with salt and pepper. Heat 2 tablespoons of oil in a large sauté pan over high heat. Cook the pork chops in batches, making sure not to overcrowd the pan. Cook for about 4 minutes on each side or until golden brown. You may need to add more oil with the remaining chops. Place the browned chops in a large baking dish.
3. Add the remaining oil to the sauté pan, set on medium heat. Add the onions and cook them slowly over medium heat until they start to brown. Sprinkle them with sugar and continue to cook, stirring, until the onions are well browned. Add the garlic and cook for 1 minute more. Arrange the onions on top of the chops and add the beef broth. The chops should be just covered with liquid. Cover the dish with foil and bake for about 45 to 60 minutes or until tender.
4. To finish the dish, remove the cover and sprinkle the cheese over the chops. Bake, uncovered, for about 7 minutes more, until the cheese is melted and golden brown. Garnish with fresh parsley.

Stuffed Bell Peppers

Serves 5
Carb Level: Moderate

Per serving:	
Carbohydrate:	18.0 g
Protein:	52.5 g

Increase the cooking times if you use the large peppers to account for the density of the filling.

10 medium-size or 5 large green bell peppers
1½ cups chopped onions
½ cup chopped carrots
3 pounds ground sirloin beef
2 tablespoons minced fresh parsley
1 tablespoon finely chopped garlic
1 teaspoon dried thyme
1 teaspoon dried basil

2 teaspoons salt
1 teaspoon freshly ground black pepper
¼ teaspoon cayenne pepper
1 tablespoon Worcestershire sauce
1 (28-ounce) can chopped tomatoes
1 cup grated Parmesan cheese

1. Preheat oven to 350°.
2. Slice off the tops of the green peppers and remove the seeds and membranes.
3. In a medium-size bowl, combine the onions, carrots, ground meat, parsley, garlic, thyme, basil, salt, pepper, cayenne, Worcestershire sauce, and tomatoes.
4. Stuff each pepper to the top with the ground beef filling. Place the peppers upright in a lightly oiled baking dish. Bake for about 55 to 60 minutes or until the beef is cooked through and the peppers are tender. When the peppers are cooked, top them with the cheese and place them back into the oven until the cheese is melted.

Beware of Additives

There are many Web sites touting comfort foods. Make sure you research the products before purchasing online. Many of the preheat-packaged products contain commercial thickeners that are high in carbohydrate.

Pot Roast with Vegetable Sauce

2 tablespoons olive oil
1 (4-pound) boneless beef sirloin
  steak
Salt and freshly ground black
  pepper to taste
1 cup thinly sliced onions
1 cup chopped celery
1 cup chopped carrots
3 teaspoons fresh thyme leaves
  or 1 teaspoon dried
Large pinch of ground allspice
Large pinch ground cloves

3 fresh flat-leaf parsley sprigs, plus
  extra, chopped, for garnish
2 bay leaves, broken in half
3 large garlic cloves, peeled and
  crushed
1 (28-ounce) can Italian-style
  tomatoes, drained and
  coarsely chopped
3 cups beef broth
2 cups dry white wine
Sugar (optional)
2 teaspoons unsalted butter

Serves 8
Carb Level: Moderate

Per serving:	
Carbohydrate:	11.1 g
Protein:	47.0 g

Serve with a vibrant green vegetable or another favorite for a change of pace from the standard potatoes and carrots.

1. Preheat oven to 350°.
2. Heat the oil in a Dutch over medium-high heat. Pat the roast dry and season with salt and pepper. Cook the roast on each side for about 5 minutes or until brown. Remove and set the roast aside.
3. In the same pan, add the onions, celery, and carrots; cook for 5 minutes, stirring, or until the vegetables are tender. Add the thyme, allspice, cloves, parsley sprigs, bay leaves, garlic, tomatoes, broth, and wine; stir to mix well. Return the roast to the pan and bring the liquid to a simmer. Transfer the contents of the pan to the oven and cook, covered, for 2½ to 3 hours or until the meat begins to fall apart. Baste and turn the roast every 30 minutes during the cooking process.
4. When the roast is done, remove the meat from the pan. Strain the vegetables from the liquid and discard the bay leaves. In a food processor, purée the vegetables until smooth. Add the puréed vegetables back to the liquid. Add a little sugar if it is too acidic.
5. Over medium-high heat, reduce the sauce by ⅓ or until it coats the back of a spoon. Season with salt and pepper and swirl in the butter.
6. To serve, cut the roast into thin slices, spoon the sauce over the top, and garnish with parsley. Serve additional sauce in a bowl to pass.

Classic Meat Loaf

Serves 6

Carb Level: Moderate

Per serving:

Carbohydrate:	15.8 g
Protein:	44.5 g

Serve with Tomato Sauce (see recipe on page 67) for a delicious hot entrée. Also good the next day sliced and eaten cold.

ॐ

4 tablespoons butter
1 cup chopped mushrooms
½ cup chopped onion
2 pounds ground beef
½ pound ground pork
½ pound ground veal
¼ cup minced fresh parsley
Salt and freshly ground black
    pepper to taste

½ cup heavy cream
1 cup bread crumbs
1 cup grated Gruyère cheese,
    divided

1. Preheat oven to 350°.
2. Melt the butter in a medium-size sauté pan over medium-high heat. When the butter starts to foam, add the mushrooms and onion; cook for about 5 minutes or until tender.
3. Transfer the sautéed vegetables to a large bowl. Add the ground meat, parsley, salt and pepper, cream, bread crumbs, and ¾ cup of the cheese; mix well, then press the mixture into a loaf pan. Sprinkle the top with the remaining cheese and bake for about 1 hour or until done.

Mashed Cauliflower?

Use cauliflower as a satisfying potato substitute: Steam the cauliflower florets until soft. Purée in a food processor until smooth. Add butter, cream or sour cream, and salt and pepper until the desired taste and consistency is achieved. Serve hot, garnished with grated cheese if desired. A ½ cup serving of cauliflower has 2.6 grams of carbohydrates.

Chicken Potpie Stew

1 pound boneless, skinless
   chicken breasts
2 cups (or more as needed)
   chicken stock
1 medium onion, diced
2 carrots, diced
2 stalks celery, diced
3 tablespoons arrowroot
½ cup evaporated skim milk

2 tablespoons chopped fresh
   parsley
1 tablespoon chopped fresh
   tarragon
Salt and freshly ground black
   pepper to taste

Serves 4
Carb Level: Moderate

Per serving:

Carbohydrate:	17.8 g
Protein:	25.2 g

A great do-ahead recipe for a group, easily prepared a day ahead and gently reheated just before serving.

1. Rinse the chicken under cold running water and pat dry on paper towels. Trim the chicken of any fat, then cut into medium dice. Place the chicken in a medium-size saucepot and add the stock. The stock should just cover the chicken. Use more if needed. Bring the liquid to a gentle simmer. Simmer until the chicken is just cooked. Remove the chicken with a slotted spoon and reserve.

2. Add the onion, carrots, and celery to the stock, and cook at a simmer until the vegetables are tender. Dilute the arrowroot in the evaporated milk and add it to the stock and vegetables. Bring the stock to a full simmer to activate the arrowroot. Remove the pot from the heat and stir in the parsley, tarragon, and salt and pepper. Return the chicken to the sauce and simmer just to heat through. Serve in warm bowls.

Chili, Chili, Chili

Modernize your chili—eliminate the beans and reduce the canned tomatoes. Add some ground New Mexican red chilies and spices such as cumin, paprika, cayenne, and oregano to develop the flavor. Add a tablespoon of cornmeal if you require a thickener. Garnish the bowls with sour cream, chopped cilantro, and grated cheeses.

CHAPTER 12
Breakfast

Strawberry Jam ❖	192
Hollandaise Sauce ❖	192
Cream Cheese and Scallion Scramble ❖	193
Steak and Eggs	194
Homemade Breakfast Sausage Patties	195
Corned Beef "Hash"	196
Scrambled Eggs with Lox and Onions ❖	197
Herbed Omelet	198
Denver Scramble ❖	199
Zucchini Frittata ❖	200
Corn and Egg Pudding ❖	201
Crabmeat Omelet	202

❖ **Indicates Easy Recipe** ❖

Strawberry Jam

Serves 10

Carb Level: Low

Per serving:

Carbohydrate:	3.7 g
Protein:	3.3 g

This jam can accompany any breakfast dish.

∾

1 pint fresh ripe strawberries
Juice of ½ lemon
¼ cup water

1¼-ounce envelope of unflavored gelatin
5 teaspoons sugar substitute or
less to taste

1. Wash, stem, and quarter the berries. In a medium-size nonreactive saucepan over medium heat, simmer the berries with the lemon juice, covered, for about 3 minutes or until the berries are soft and start to release their juices.
2. In a small bowl, pour the water over the gelatin and allow to soften for 1 minute. Add this to the berries and remove from the heat. Mix in the sugar substitute to taste and store covered in the refrigerator. Serve when completely chilled.

Hollandaise Sauce

Serves 6

Carb Level: Low

Per serving:

Carbohydrate:	0.6 g
Protein:	1.6 g

This is a classic match with any egg dish. Add tarragon for a variation of flavors.

∾

½ cup butter
3 egg yolks
2 tablespoons fresh-squeezed
lemon juice

Dash of cayenne pepper
Salt and freshly ground black
pepper to taste

Melt the butter in a small saucepan over low heat. In a blender, mix the egg yolks, lemon juice, and cayenne. With the motor running, add the melted butter in a slow stream. Blend for about 30 seconds or until thick. Keep over a bowl of very hot water, stirring occasionally until ready to serve. Add salt and pepper to taste.

Cream Cheese and Scallion Scramble

3 tablespoons unsalted butter
2/3 cup scallions, minced
1 tablespoon shallots, minced
10 large eggs
4 ounces cream cheese, cut
   into bits and softened

Salt and freshly ground black
   pepper to taste
1 tablespoon snipped fresh dill
Chopped chives or scallion
   tops, thinly sliced for
   garnish

Serves 4

Carb Level: Low

Per serving:	
Carbohydrate:	3.3 g
Protein:	15.1 g

This is a simple recipe
that kids also enjoy.

1. Melt the butter in a medium-size nonstick sauté pan over medium heat. When the butter starts to foam, add the scallions and shallots; cook for about 2 minutes or until the scallions are tender.
2. In a bowl, whisk together the eggs, cream cheese, salt and pepper, and dill. Pour the mixture into the sauté pan and cook over low heat, stirring, until cooked. Transfer to a plate and garnish with chopped chives or scallions.

Does Color Matter?

Is there a difference between brown-shelled eggs and white-shelled eggs? The shell color does not affect the nutritional value, cooking characteristics, or quality. Egg shell color is determined by the breed of the chicken.

Steak and Eggs

Serves 4
Carb Level: Low

Per serving:	
Carbohydrate:	1.2 g
Protein:	33.2 g

If you don't own a cast iron skillet, use the heaviest ovenproof sauté pan you have.

1 tablespoon canola oil
1-pound sirloin steak (about
  1 inch thick)
Salt and cayenne pepper
2 tablespoons butter

8 large eggs
1 teaspoon snipped chives

1. Preheat oven to 350°.
2. Preheat a large cast iron skillet over medium heat until hot, about 5 minutes. Raise the heat to high and add the oil. Season the steak with salt and cayenne pepper. Place the steak in the skillet and cook on each side for about 4 minutes or until golden brown. Transfer the steak to the oven and cook for about 5 minutes for medium-rare.
3. Let the steak rest, tented with tin foil, for 10 minutes.
4. Heat 2 nonstick sauté pans over medium-low heat. Melt 1 tablespoon of butter in each pan. Break 4 eggs into each sauté pan. Season the eggs lightly with the chives, salt, and cayenne pepper. Cook until the whites are just set. Divide the eggs among 4 warm plates.
5. Cut the steak into slices and serve with the eggs.

Food Safety Tip
Salmonella bacteria does not come from the shell or cracks in the shell, but from the yolk itself. You can have a perfectly clean, crack-free egg that contains salmonella.

Homemade
Breakfast Sausage Patties

1 pound lean ground pork
¼ cup bread crumbs
2 tablespoons cream
2 teaspoons pure maple syrup
2 teaspoons grated orange zest
2 teaspoons finely chopped
  fresh parsley
⅛ teaspoon dried sage
½ teaspoon red pepper flakes

½ teaspoon salt
½ teaspoon freshly ground
  black pepper
1½ tablespoons canola oil

Serves 6
Carb Level: Low

Per serving:

Carbohydrate:	5.4 g
Protein:	20.2 g

You can omit the maple syrup and add your own blend of herbs or spices.

ॐ

1. In a medium-size bowl, use your hands to mix together all of the ingredients until completely bended. Divide into 12 equal portions.
2. Place a nonstick sauté pan over medium heat. Wearing plastic gloves, gently form each patty about ½-inch thick and 2 inches in diameter. Working in batches, cook the patties on each side for about 5 minutes or until they are golden brown. (Make sure they are cooked all the way through.) Serve immediately.

Sausage Fact
Nutritional information: ¼ pound of breakfast sausage equals 1.2 grams of carbohydrates and 13.3 grams of protein.

Corned Beef "Hash"

Serves 4	
Carb Level: Low	
Per serving:	
Carbohydrate:	6.1 g
Protein:	26.3 g

Serve a poached egg on top of the hash for an amazing breakfast.

∾

2 tablespoons unsalted butter

1 large mild yellow onion, cut into $^1/_2$-inch dice

1 red bell pepper, seeded, trimmed, and cut into $^1/_2$-inch dice

$1^1/_2$ pounds unsliced cooked lean corned beef, cut into $^1/_4$-inch dice

$^1/_3$ cup milk

$^1/_2$ cup finely chopped fresh parsley

2 tablespoons finely chopped fresh chives

Salt and freshly ground black pepper to taste

4 tablespoons vegetable oil, divided

1. Melt the butter in a large nonstick sauté pan over medium heat. Add the onion and pepper and cook for about 5 minutes or until tender. Transfer the vegetables to a large bowl and set aside.

2. Add the corned beef, milk, parsley, chives, and salt and pepper to the vegetables; toss well to mix.

3. Heat 2 tablespoons of the oil in the sauté pan over medium heat. Add the hash mixture, pressing it down with the back of a spatula to form an even compact cake. Reduce the heat to medium-low and cook for about 15 minutes, shaking the pan occasionally, or until the bottom is golden brown and crusty. Transfer the patty to a heatproof plate.

4. Heat the remaining 2 tablespoons of oil in the same pan and slide the hash cake, browned side up, back into the pan. Cook the second side for about 10 minutes or until golden brown and crusty. Transfer onto the same heatproof plate and cut into wedges.

Scrambled Eggs
with Lox and Onions

2 tablespoons butter
½ sweet onion, finely chopped
12 eggs, lightly beaten
6 ounces lox, thinly sliced and
    cut into 1-inch-long, ¼-inch-
    wide strips

Freshly ground black pepper
    to taste
1 tablespoon finely chopped
    fresh chives for garnish

Serves 6
Carb Level: Low

Per serving:	
Carbohydrate:	2.0 g
Protein:	17.8 g

This is an easy break-
fast dish to prepare
when guests are over.

1. Melt the butter in a nonstick sauté pan over medium-low heat.
   Add the onion and cook for about 4 minutes until slightly brown.
2. Add the eggs and raise the heat. Stir occasionally while the eggs
   cook. While the eggs are still fairly loose, add the lox and pepper.
   Continue stirring until the eggs are cooked to your liking.
3. Serve on warm plates and garnish with chopped chives.

Taking Medication?

*Some medications will reduce your body's ability to absorb and
use certain vitamins and minerals. Periodically review your diet plan
and medications with your doctor to see if a supplement is needed.
Always review your overall plan with your doctor whenever you
implement a change in either diet, medication, supplements, or exer-
cise plans.*

Herbed Omelet

Serves 1
Carb Level: Low

Per serving:

Carbohydrate:	2.4 g
Protein:	19.2 g

Adding grated cheese when you add the herbs lends even more flavor to this dish.

∾

3 eggs
Salt and freshly ground black
  pepper to taste
1 tablespoon butter

1 teaspoon each finely
  chopped: fresh flat-leaf
  parsley, fresh chives, fresh
  chervil, fresh tarragon

1. In a medium-size bowl, whisk together the eggs, and salt and pepper until frothy.
2. Melt the butter in a small nonstick sauté pan over medium heat. Add the eggs and, as they begin to set, use a spatula to carefully lift the edges and gently push them toward the center, tilting the pan slightly to allow the liquid egg on top to flow underneath. Continue to cook the eggs until they are almost set but still slightly moist on top.
3. Sprinkle the herbs over the surface of the eggs. Carefully slide the omelet from the pan to a warm plate and, when halfway out, flip the pan over to fold the omelet in half. Serve immediately.

Ethnic Variations

Many combinations of herbs will work with this recipe. Try cilantro with a touch of minced jalapeños for a Mexican flair and top with homemade salsa—or try basil with a touch of oregano for an Italian flavor and top with Tomato Sauce (see recipe on page 67).

Denver Scramble

2 tablespoons unsalted butter

½ yellow onion, cut into ½-inch dice

½ green bell pepper, seeded and cut into ½-inch squares

½ red bell pepper, seeded and cut into ½-inch squares

6 ounces Canadian bacon, cut into ½-inch dice

8 eggs, lightly beaten

Salt and freshly ground white pepper to taste

2 ounces Cheddar cheese, shredded

1 tablespoon finely chopped fresh parsley

Serves 4
Carb Level: Low

Per serving:

Carbohydrate:	5.0 g
Protein:	25.3 g

Cleanup is easy with this recipe since everything is done in 1 pan.

1. Melt the butter in a medium-size nonstick sauté pan over medium heat. Add the onion and peppers, and cook for about 3 minutes or until tender. Add the Canadian bacon and cook for 1 more minute.
2. Add the eggs to the pan and season with salt and pepper. Cook at medium-low heat, stirring frequently. Stir in the cheese and continue cooking until done to your liking.
3. Serve on warm plates and garnish with parsley.

Juice Alert

Note the high carb counts for just 1 cup of fresh-squeezed juices:

Orange Juice	25.8 g
Grapefruit Juice	22.7 g
Cranberry Juice	36.4 g
Lemonade	26.9 g

Zucchini Frittata

Serves 6

Carb Level: Low

Per serving:

Carbohydrate:	4.5 g
Protein:	13.5 g

Goes great with Tomato Sauce (see page 67).

⌒

1½ pounds small zucchini
10 eggs
¼ cup freshly grated
*   Parmesan cheese, divided*
Salt and freshly ground black
*   pepper to taste*

2 tablespoons unsalted butter
2 tablespoons olive oil

1. Preheat oven to 350°.
2. Trim the zucchini and cut it crosswise into very thin slices. In a medium-size bowl, beat the eggs until light and frothy. Add the zucchini, half of the cheese, and the salt and pepper.
3. Melt the butter and add the oil to a medium-size nonstick ovenproof sauté pan over medium heat. Add the egg mixture. Sprinkle with the remaining cheese. Place it in the oven and bake until set but still slightly moist, about 20 minutes.
4. Serve the frittata directly from the pan or slide it onto a plate. Cut into wedges and serve immediately.

Egg Facts
1 whole large egg equals 0.6 grams of carbohydrates and 6.3 grams of protein. The breakdown: 1 large egg yolk equals 0.3 grams of carbohydrates and 2.8 grams of protein; 1 large egg white equals 0.3 grams of carbohydrates and 2.8 grams of protein.

Corn and Egg Pudding

Butter, for greasing
2 whole eggs
2 egg yolks
2½ cups fresh corn kernels
½ cup heavy cream
¼ pound smoked ham,
   chopped

¼ pound Gruyère cheese,
   shredded
½ teaspoon sweet paprika

Serves 6
Carb Level: Moderate

Per serving:	
Carbohydrate:	13.2 g
Protein:	11.2 g

You can substitute canned creamed corn if fresh is not available.

1. Preheat oven to 375°. Butter a small baking dish.
2. In a bowl, whisk together the eggs and the yolks until blended. Stir in the corn and cream until well mixed. Stir in the ham, cheese, and paprika.
3. Pour the mixture into the prepared baking dish. Bake for about 30 minutes or until lightly golden. Scoop out onto warm plates and serve immediately.

 Milk It for All It's Worth

Note the following carb counts for 1 cup of milk:

1% Soy Milk	4.3 g
1% Cow's Milk	11.7 g
Whole Cow's Milk	11.4 g

Crabmeat Omelet

Serves 1
Carb Level: Low

Per serving:

Carbohydrate:	1.9 g
Protein:	24.8 g

For a more indulgent dish, top the omelet with Hollandaise or Tomato Sauce (see recipes on pages 192 and 67).

3 eggs
¼ teaspoon salt
Pinch freshly ground white pepper
1½ tablespoons unsalted butter, divided
2 ounces flaked cooked crabmeat
¼ teaspoon grated lemon zest
Fresh dill sprigs or chopped parsley for garnish

1. In a medium-size bowl, whisk together the eggs, salt, and pepper until frothy.
2. Melt ½ tablespoon of the butter in a small nonstick sauté pan over low heat. Add the crabmeat and cook until just heated through. Stir in the lemon zest. Cover to keep warm and set aside.
3. Melt the remaining butter in another small nonstick sauté pan over medium heat. Add the eggs. As they begin to set, use a spatula to carefully lift the edges and gently push them toward the center, tilting the pan slightly to allow the liquid egg on top to flow underneath. Continue to cook the eggs until they are almost set.
4. Sprinkle the crabmeat over half of the omelet. When sliding the omelet out of the pan, start with the crab-covered side toward the plate. When the omelet is halfway out, flip the pan over to fold the omelet in half. Garnish with dill or parsley.

Glazed Bananas	204
Orange Cups with Lemon Cream	205
Warm Berry Compote ❖	206
Champagne-Marinated Summer Berries ❖	206
Chocolate Grand Marnier Mousse	207
Chocolate Meringue Cookies	208
Chocolate Fudge ❖	209
Egg Custard ❖	209
Refrigerator Pumpkin Pie with Macadamia Nut Crust	210
Vanilla Ice Cream	211
Blanc Manger ❖	212
No-Crust Cheesecake	213
Mocha Mousse	214
Rhubarb and Strawberry Cream	215

❖ **Indicates Easy Recipe** ❖

Glazed Bananas

Serves 6

Carb Level: Moderate

Per serving:

Carbohydrate:	19.8 g
Protein:	1.5 g

The banana slices can be prepared ahead of time and baked just before serving.

❧

$^{1}/_{2}$ cup crumbs of sugar-free
   butter cookies
2 teaspoons canola oil
1 teaspoon butter, melted
1 large egg white
2 tablespoons honey

1 teaspoon fresh-squeezed
   lemon juice
3 large ripe, but firm, bananas
Lemon wedges for garnish
Mint sprigs for garnish

1. Preheat oven to 450°. Line a baking sheet with aluminum foil. Set a baking rack on top and coat it with nonstick cooking spray.
2. In a shallow dish, combine the cookie crumbs, oil, and butter. Mix with your fingertips until well blended; set aside.
3. In a medium-size bowl, whisk together the egg white, honey, and lemon juice; set aside.
4. Peel the bananas and trim the pointed tips. Cut the bananas crosswise into $^{3}/_{4}$-inch pieces. Dip each banana piece into the egg-white mixture, then transfer them to the crumb mixture. Roll the banana pieces in the crumbs, trying to lightly but evenly coat them. (It helps to use dinner forks to transfer the bananas during the coating process.) Place the bananas on the prepared baking rack.
5. Bake the bananas until crisp, golden, and heated through, about 8 to 12 minutes. Arrange the hot bananas on dessert plates, garnish with lemon wedges and mint sprigs, and serve with Vanilla Ice Cream (see recipe on page 211).

Avoid Temptation

Clean your pantry, kitchen shelves, and cabinets of high-carb products that you will not be using. Donate unopened usable items to your local homeless shelter. Call the shelter before dropping off the food to find out the proper procedure for donations.

Orange Cups with Lemon Cream

4 large oranges
Grated zest of 1 lemon
⅓ cup light whipping cream
½ cup vanilla yogurt

Julienne strips of lemon and
*   orange peel for garnish*

Serves 6
Carb Level: Moderate

Per serving:	
Carbohydrate:	11.6 g
Protein:	2.2 g

This dish must be served the same day it's prepared, or the filling will start to separate.

1. With a sharp knife, cut each orange in half crosswise. Remove the flesh (with the help of a grapefruit spoon) and chop finely, then place in a bowl. Set the peels aside.
2. Mix the lemon zest with the chopped orange flesh. In a separate bowl, whip the cream until it is stiff. With a rubber spatula, fold the yogurt into the whipped cream. Add the cream mixture to the chopped oranges, and stir gently to mix. Very thinly slice the bottom off each orange shell so they sit level on a plate.
3. Fill all the shells with the orange mixture, then place on a serving plate. Refrigerate the filled shells until ready to serve. To serve, decorate with lemon and orange peels strips.

Desserts on the Web

There are a number of new Web sites offering low-carb sweets. Try the following sites to purchase premade sugar-free desserts and products: www.lowcarbmart.com *and* www.locarbdiner.com.

Warm Berry Compote

Serves 6

Carb Level: Moderate

Per serving:

Carbohydrate:	12.9 g
Protein:	0.7 g

A great recipe in winter when you want the flavor of fresh berries. Frozen berries are put to perfect use in this cooked berry recipe.

4 cups assorted frozen berries, no sugar added, thawed

¼ teaspoon (or to taste) sugar substitute

½ cup butter

1. Simmer the berries with about 2 tablespoons of water in a nonreactive medium-size saucepan for about 5 minutes. Add a pinch of sugar substitute, check for flavor, add more sugar substitute as desired. Add the butter and stir in to combine.
2. Remove the pan from the heat, stir 1 more time, and divide the compote among 6 small bowls. Top with Vanilla Ice Cream (see recipe on page 211) or whipped heavy cream.

Champagne-Marinated Summer Berries

Serves 4

Carb Level: Moderate

Per serving:

Carbohydrate:	16.5 g
Protein:	0.9 g

Add the sugar substitute pinch by pinch until you determine the natural sweetness of the berries.

1 cup strawberries, hulled and cut in half

1 cup raspberries

½ cup red currants

½ cup blueberries

Sugar substitute to taste

¼ cup fresh lemon juice

1 cup chilled champagne

Mint sprigs for garnish

1. Mix all the berries in a glass bowl and sprinkle them with a pinch of sugar substitute and half of the lemon juice; set aside for 10 minutes.
2. To serve, spoon the fruit into glass dishes. At the table, pour the chilled champagne over the fruit and decorate with mint sprigs.

Chocolate Grand Marnier Mousse

4 ounces unsweetened chocolate, roughly chopped
4 eggs, separated
¼ cup Grand Marnier
¼ cup brandy

½ cup heavy cream, whipped
Pinch of salt

<table>
<tr><td colspan="2">Serves 6</td></tr>
<tr><td colspan="2">Carb Level: Low</td></tr>
<tr><td colspan="2">Per serving:</td></tr>
<tr><td>Carbohydrate:</td><td>10.0 g</td></tr>
<tr><td>Protein:</td><td>6.5 g</td></tr>
</table>

This dessert is very rich, so servings should be kept small.

1. Melt the chocolate by placing it in a bowl over a saucepan of simmering water until it melts (do not let the water touch the bowl filled with chocolate). Put the egg yolks into another bowl and pour the melted chocolate over them; whisk to blend thoroughly. Add the Grand Marnier, brandy, and cream; mix thoroughly.
2. In a separate bowl, beat the egg whites with the salt until medium peaks form. With a rubber spatula, fold this mixture in thirds, very slowly and carefully, into the chocolate cream so that it is completely combined but still light and fluffy.
3. Spoon into individual ramekins and refrigerate for 2 hours before serving.

Elegant End
End a meal with ¼ perfectly ripe pear, cored, sliced, and fanned on an attractive plate, served with 2 ounces of a fine cheese such as an imported French Muenster or English Stilton (8.3 grams carbohydrates).

Chocolate Meringue Cookies

<table>
<tr><td colspan="2">Serves 12</td></tr>
<tr><td colspan="2">Carb Level: Moderate</td></tr>
<tr><td colspan="2">Per serving:</td></tr>
<tr><td>Carbohydrate:</td><td>13.3 g</td></tr>
<tr><td>Protein:</td><td>1.1 g</td></tr>
</table>

You can make "petite" cookies by using a teaspoon measure of batter instead of a tablespoon.

ॐ

3 large eggs, separated
⅛ teaspoon cream of tartar
¾ cup granulated sugar

3 tablespoons unsweetened
cocoa powder, plus extra
for garnish

1. Preheat the oven to 375°. Cover 2 baking sheets with parchment paper.
2. Place the egg whites and cream of tartar in a medium-size bowl or the bowl of an electric mixer; mix on medium-high speed until soft peaks form. Gradually beat in the granulated sugar (1 tablespoon at a time) until the whites are stiff and shiny.
3. Sift the cocoa over the egg whites and gently fold in until just blended. Drop tablespoons of the batter 1 inch apart on the prepared baking sheets. Bake for 30 to 35 minutes, until the cookies are dry. Carefully peel the cookies from the paper and cool on a wire rack. When cool, sprinkle the cookies with a little more cocoa powder. Store, covered, at room temperature.

A Sophisticated Dessert

Tradition dictates that dessert, or the ending course of a formal meal, include a sweet, carbohydrate-heavy dessert. Consider ending the meal in the European style by focusing on a sophisticated cheese course for the final course with a very simple dessert, such as a small platter of petite cookies for those desiring something sweet.

Chocolate Fudge

1 cup heavy cream
8 ounces unsweetened choco-
    late, chopped
1 3/4 cups sugar substitute,
    granular style
2 tablespoons unsalted butter
1 tablespoon vanilla extract

Line a baking sheet with waxed paper or parchment paper. Spray with nonstick coating. Place a medium-size saucepan over medium heat and add the cream. Bring to a boil, add the chocolate, and stir until completely melted. Remove the pan from the heat and add the sugar substitute, butter, and vanilla extract. Mix until smooth and thoroughly combined. Transfer to the prepared baking sheet. Spread evenly over the entire sheet. Refrigerate until cool and stiff, about 2 hours. To serve, cut the fudge into squares.

Serves 40

Carb Level: Low

Per serving:

Carbohydrate:	2.0 g
Protein:	0.8 g

The quality of the chocolate is key; purchase quality imported chocolate if available.

Egg Custard

3 large eggs
4 packets sugar substitute
1/4 teaspoon salt
2 cups milk
1/4 teaspoon vanilla extract
1/8 teaspoon grated nutmeg
1/8 teaspoon ground cinnamon
Fresh raspberries for garnish
    (optional)

Preheat oven to 350°. Beat the eggs in a large mixing bowl until frothy and blended. Add the sugar substitute and salt; mix to combine. Add the milk, vanilla, nutmeg, and cinnamon; mix well to combine. Divide the mixture into six ramekins or other custard cups. Set the filled cups in a large baking dish and add enough boiling water to fill the dish with 1 inch of water. Bake until the custard is set (doesn't jiggle if shaken with a pair of tongs), about 30 minutes. Serve warm, room temperature, or chilled, with a garnish of fresh raspberries on top.

Serves 6

Carb Level: Low

Per serving:

Carbohydrate:	4.9 g
Protein:	5.8 g

Try orange extract instead of the vanilla extract and add a touch of grated orange zest for a delicious orange custard.

Refrigerator Pumpkin Pie
with Macadamia Nut Crust

<table>
<tr><td>Serves 8</td></tr>
<tr><td>Carb Level: Moderate</td></tr>
</table>

Per serving:

Carbohydrate:	10.8 g
Protein:	3.4 g

A delicious do-ahead dessert—this recipe requires a few mixing bowls but is worth the effort.

∾

1½ cups finely chopped macadamia nuts
16 packets sugar substitute
2 tablespoons butter, softened, plus extra for greasing
1 packet gelatin
¼ cup water
1 teaspoon pumpkin pie spice
1 (15-ounce) can pumpkin purée
2 teaspoons grated orange zest
1½ cups heavy cream
2 teaspoons vanilla extract

1. Heat oven to 400°. Butter the bottom and sides of a 9-inch spring-form pan.
2. In a medium-size bowl, combine the macadamia nuts, 4 packets of sugar substitute, and butter; mix well. Press the mixture onto the bottom and 1 inch up the sides of the prepared pan. Bake for 10 minutes, until golden brown. Cool on a wire rack.
3. In a small bowl, sprinkle the gelatin over the water; let sit for 5 minutes until the gelatin softens. Heat a small skillet over medium heat and toast the pumpkin pie spice for 1 to 2 minutes, until fragrant, stirring frequently. Reduce heat to low, stir in the gelatin mixture, and cook 1 to 2 minutes until the gelatin melts. Remove from heat and cool to room temperature.
4. Place the pumpkin purée in a large bowl and mash with a fork to loosen. Mix in the orange zest. In another large bowl, using an electric mixer on high speed, beat the cream with the remaining 12 packets of sugar substitute and the vanilla until soft peaks form. With a rubber spatula, slowly fold in the gelatin mixture (if too stiff, heat on the stove until melted but not hot). In 3 parts, gently fold the whipped cream mixture into the pumpkin purée. Pour the filling into the cooled pie shell and smooth the top. Refrigerate at least 3 hours before serving.

Vanilla Ice Cream

1 quart heavy cream
6 egg yolks
1 quart whole milk
1 cup Equal Spoonful

½ teaspoon salt
2 tablespoons vanilla extract
3 egg whites

Serves 12
Carb Level: Low

Per serving:	
Carbohydrate:	6.9 g
Protein:	5.7 g

You don't have to have an ice cream machine to make this!

❧

1. Oil a 9" × 5" metal bread loaf pan. Line the pan with 2 layers of plastic wrap, leaving at least a 4-inch overhang on the long sides. Freeze the pan for 30 minutes.

2. Using an electric mixer, whip the heavy cream until it thickens, but is still somewhat loose (before soft peaks form). Beat in the egg yolks, whole milk, sweetener, salt, and vanilla until the mixture is not quite as thick as regular whipped cream.

3. In a separate bowl, beat the egg whites until they hold soft peaks. Fold the egg whites into the whipped mixture until uniformly blended. (If you have an ice cream machine, add the mixture to the prepared machine following the manufacturer's instructions.) Pour the mixture into the chilled pan, cover with foil, and freeze for 12 to 24 hours until solid.

4. Place your food processor bowl and blade in the freezer. Dip the metal loaf pan into hot water for 5 seconds to ease in removing the plastic-wrapped ice cream. Firmly pull up on the plastic wrap and remove the ice cream loaf. Peel off the plastic wrap. Cut the loaf into thick slices with a large knife, slicing off only the amount desired to be served. Cut each slice into 4 chunks, immediately put these chunks into the chilled food processor bowl, and begin to process in 5-second pulses, adding as little milk or cream as needed to make the ice cream smooth. Scrape down the sides of the bowl as necessary. Serve immediately when the ice cream is smooth in texture or freeze to hold for several minutes if serving as an accompaniment to another dessert.

Blanc Manger

Serves 6
Carb Level: Low

Per serving:	
Carbohydrate:	5.1 g
Protein:	2.6 g

A very lovely, elegant, and classic French dessert.

∾

Cooking spray, for greasing
1 envelope gelatin
2 cups heavy cream
8 packets sugar substitute
½ teaspoon almond extract
1 vanilla bean
½ cup fresh berries
(any kind) for garnish

1. Lightly spray six ramekins or custard cups with cooking spray. In a small bowl, sprinkle the gelatin over 3 tablespoons cold water; let stand for 5 minutes until softened.
2. Combine the cream, ½ cup water, the sweetener, almond extract, and vanilla bean in a medium-size saucepan; bring to a boil over medium heat. Remove from heat, add the gelatin mixture, and stir until melted.
3. Pour the mixture into the prepared cups. Cover surface with plastic wrap to prevent skin from forming. Refrigerate for at least 3 hours. When ready to serve, score a small sharp knife along the sides of the ramekin to separate the custard from the dish. Turn out onto serving platters or individual plates and serve with a few fresh berries.

Little Nibbles

Consider serving a small platter of sweet nibbles instead of full servings of a rich carbohydrate-laden dessert. Chocolate-covered roasted coffee beans are elegant treats, Australian candied ginger pieces, chocolate covered nuts, and nut meringues are also nice finishes.

No-Crust Cheesecake

1 tablespoon butter, for
   greasing
2 pounds cream cheese, at
   room temperature
1 cup sugar substitute
4 large eggs, at room
   temperature

¼ teaspoon orange extract
¼ teaspoon lemon extract
2 tablespoons heavy cream
1 teaspoon pure vanilla extract

Serves 12	
Carb Level: Moderate	
Per serving:	
Carbohydrate:	13.4 g
Protein:	7.9 g

You can vary the flavor by substituting different extracts for the citrus extracts, but always add the vanilla extract.

∾

1. Preheat oven to 350°. Butter the bottom and sides of a 9-inch spring-form pan and set aside.
2. Using an electric mixer, beat the cream cheese on medium speed until it's very smooth. Slowly beat in the sweetener 1 tablespoon at a time. Then, add the eggs 1 at a time, beating well after each addition. Add the remaining ingredients, scrape down the bowl, and stir to combine.
3. Pour the cheesecake batter into the prepared spring-form pan and smooth the top with a rubber spatula. Bake for 10 minutes. Turn down the heat to 275° and bake for approximately 1 hour, or until the edges are lightly brown (the cheesecake may be cracked on top). Turn off the oven.
4. Remove the cheesecake from the oven, run a thin-bladed knife around the edge of the pan, and return the pan to the oven to cool slowly. If the center of the cheesecake still looks a little undercooked, it will firm up in the oven as it slowly cooks.
5. Cover the cooled cheesecake with the plastic wrap and refrigerate overnight, or up to 3 days. To serve, run a knife around the edges again and remove the sides of the spring-form pan.

Mocha Mousse

Serves 6

Carb Level: Moderate

Per serving:

Carbohydrate:	12.6 g
Protein:	5.0 g

Don't overmix the mousse when adding the chocolate to the egg whites.

～

4 ounces semisweet chocolate, cut into small chunks

4 large eggs, separated

1 teaspoon vanilla extract

2 teaspoons brewed strong black coffee or instant espresso, cooled

Pinch of salt

1. Put the chocolate in a stainless steel bowl and place the bowl over the top of a saucepot of simmering water; stir until fully melted. Remove from heat and let chocolate stand for 5 minutes.
2. In a small bowl, beat the egg yolks with the vanilla extract and cooled coffee; stir into the melted chocolate, whisking well. Beat the egg whites with the salt until they form stiff peaks. Using a rubber spatula, gently fold half of the chocolate mixture into the egg whites. Fold in the remaining mixture. Fold to just blend; the mixture may appear streaky.
3. Pour into 6 ramekins, small dessert bowls, or glasses, cover, and chill for at least 4 hours or overnight.

What's the Best Way to Crack an Egg?

Hit the egg firmly, but not forcefully against a hard, flat surface. The shell shatters less so there is less chance bits of shell will be in the eggs.

Rhubarb and Strawberry Cream

4 cups diced rhubarb
11 packets sugar substitute
Pinch of salt

1 pint strawberries, cut into
small pieces, plus extra
for garnish
1 pint heavy cream

Serves 8
Carb Level: Low

Per serving:	
Carbohydrate:	8.3 g
Protein:	2.0 g

The season for fresh rhubarb is short—peak growing periods are April through June.

1. Put the diced rhubarb into a medium-size nonreactive saucepan and stew it gently, uncovered. You may need to add a tablespoon of water. Add 9 packets of sugar substitute and salt. Cook until the rhubarb is very tender and can be mashed easily with a fork. Add additional water, tablespoon by tablespoon to prevent the rhubarb from scorching. Add the strawberries and cook just until combined with the rhubarb mixture, about 4 minutes. Cool the mixture in the refrigerator for about 1 hour.
2. Whip the cream until stiff peaks have formed. Mix in the remaining 2 packets of sugar substitute. Using a rubber spatula, gently fold the whipped cream into the rhubarb mixture. Spoon the mousse into individual ramekins, cover with plastic wrap, and chill thoroughly before serving. Serve with a garnish of fresh strawberries.

A Simple Finish When Berries Are in Season

Combine ⅓ cup sliced strawberries (3.5 grams of carbohydrates), 1 teaspoon honey (5.8 grams of carbohydrates), and ¼ cup vanilla yogurt (2.6 grams of carbohydrates) for an easy and delicious treat.

Seared Salmon Carpaccio ❖	218
Smoked Salmon Rillette ❖	219
Spinach and Ricotta Filling ❖	219
Grilled Lobster with Lemon and Tarragon	220
Spring Lamb Chops	221
Roast Pheasant with Cabbage	222
Grilled Red Snapper with Basil Aioli ❖	223
White Wine–Poached Salmon ❖	224
Chutney-Glazed Smoked Ham ❖	225
Pesto-Baked Chicken ❖	226
Pork Roast ❖	227
Roasted Vidalia Onions ❖	228
Pork Crown Roast	229
Cod Cakes	230
Grilled Mushrooms and Peppers ❖	231
Coriander-Crusted Flank Steak ❖	232
Boneless Chicken Thighs with Major Grey's Chutney	233
Sautéed Ham with Cider Reduction	234
Barbecued Beef ❖	235
Sautéed Swordfish in a White Wine Sauce	236

Grilled Mediterranean Grouper	237
Cauliflower Vichyssoise ❖	238
Beef Tenderloin with Belgian Endive	239
Fish Stew	240
Venison Medallions with a Cranberry Dijon Chutney	241
Roasted Eggplant Napoleon with Marinated Goat Cheese	242
Fried Green Tomatoes ❖	243
Baked Cod with Tomatoes, Capers, and Sautéed Spinach	244
Artichoke, Cucumber, and Tomato Salad ❖	245
Roasted Rabbit with Garlic	246
Roasted Grouper with Tomatoes ❖	247
Veal Saltimboca	248
Marinated Grilled Steak Strips	250
Grilled Swordfish with Olive Tapenade	251
Pecan-Crusted Catfish with Wilted Greens ❖	252
Roasted Salmon with Goat Cheese and Tarragon	253
Mussels Steamed in White Wine ❖	254

❖ Indicates Easy Recipe ❖

Seared Salmon Carpaccio

Serves 4
Carb Level: Low

Per serving:

Carbohydrate:	6.5 g
Protein:	26.2 g

An elegant starter course for a summer dinner party. Keep the salmon chilled until you serve it.

❧

1 pound sushi-grade salmon fillet

Salt and freshly ground black pepper to taste

4 tablespoons, plus 1 teaspoon extra-virgin olive oil

2 tablespoons, plus 1 teaspoon fresh-squeezed lime juice

2 cups stemmed baby organic arugula leaves

4 ounces domestic mushrooms, trimmed and thinly sliced

1 tablespoon finely minced chives

1. Season the salmon with the salt and black pepper. Heat a heavy-bottomed, nonstick sauté pan over high heat until almost smoking. Quickly sear the top side of the salmon, only about 1 minute, then sear the other side for about 1 minute. Immediately transfer the salmon to a plate and refrigerate for 1 hour. Using a sharp knife, slice the salmon as thinly as possible. (The slices should be so thin that you should be able to see through them.) Cut enough salmon to cover the bases of 4 small chilled salad plates. Cover with plastic wrap and refrigerate.

2. In a small bowl, whisk together 3 tablespoons of the olive oil, 1 tablespoon of the lime juice, and season with salt and pepper. Toss the arugula and the mushrooms in a separate bowl and drizzle with the vinaigrette.

3. Uncover the plates of salmon and drizzle each plate with the remaining lime juice and olive oil. Sprinkle the salmon with the chives. Garnish the center of each plate with the arugula and mushrooms. Serve immediately.

The Perfect Addition to Brunch

Smoked salmon is actually a carbohydrate-free food, deliciously rich. Traditional pairings are sour cream (1.2 grams of carbohydrates per ounce), cucumber slices (1.5 grams of carbohydrates per 2 ounces), fresh dill (0.3 grams of carbohydrates per ½ teaspoon), and capers, a carbohydrate-free item.

Smoked Salmon Rillette

1 pound smoked salmon
Salt and freshly ground white
  pepper to taste
1 tablespoon unsalted butter,
  softened
2 tablespoons mayonnaise
Grated zest of 1 lemon

Juice of ½ lemon, or more
  to taste
1 tablespoon chopped dill
1 tablespoon finely minced
  fresh chives

In a food processor or blender, purée the smoked salmon, salt, and pepper until smooth. Transfer to a mixing bowl and add the butter; mix until thoroughly blended. Add the mayonnaise, lemon zest, lemon juice, dill, and chives. Add the salt and pepper and more lemon juice if desired. Cover and refrigerate for at least 2 hours.

Serves 8	
Carb Level: Low	
Per serving:	
Carbohydrate:	0.3 g
Protein:	10.5 g

Rillettes refer to "potted meat." Try this recipe as a filling for crepes.

❧

Spinach and Ricotta Filling

6 ounces frozen chopped
  spinach, thawed and drained
1 tablespoon unsalted butter
Pinch of freshly grated nutmeg

Salt and freshly ground black
  pepper to taste
1 cup ricotta cheese
1 large egg

1. In a medium-size sauté pan over medium heat, cook the spinach with the butter, nutmeg, and salt and pepper. Drain well and cool.
2. Squeeze any water out of the spinach until very dry. Mix the spinach with the ricotta and egg. Adjust seasoning as needed.

Serves 2	
Carb Level: Low	
Per serving:	
Carbohydrate:	8.1 g
Protein:	20.3 g

A very versatile and traditional filling—use for stuffed chicken breasts or as a filling for crepes.

❧

Grilled Lobster
with Lemon and Tarragon

Serves 2
Carb Level: Low

Per serving:

Carbohydrate:	2.6 g
Protein:	28.7 g

This is a perfectly elegant dish suited for an anniversary.

∾

½ cup butter
2 tablespoons fresh lemon
   juice
1½ teaspoons grated lemon
   zest
2 tablespoons chopped chives
1 tablespoon chopped fresh
   tarragon

Salt and freshly ground black
   pepper to taste
2 frozen uncooked lobster tails,
   thawed

1. Prepare a charcoal grill or preheat a gas grill to high heat.
2. In a small saucepan over low heat, melt the butter and add the lemon juice, lemon zest, chives, tarragon, and salt and pepper; set aside and keep warm.
3. Use heavy kitchen shears to split the lobster tails by cutting the length of the underside. Brush the cut side of the tails with 1 tablespoon of the butter sauce.
4. Grill the lobsters, cut-side down, for about 4 minutes. Turn them and grill for another 4 minutes. Turn them again to the cut side and grill until the lobster meat is just opaque but still juicy, about 2 minutes. Transfer to plates. Brush the lobster with the butter sauce and serve the remaining sauce in a small ramekin on the side.

Serving Lobster Graciously

Provide your guests with a clean towel and small bowl of warm water with a floating lemon slice for use as a finger bowl. Another alternative is to remove the meat from the shell before serving. Use kitchen shears to split the shell. Brush the meat with the seasoned butter before serving.

Spring Lamb Chops

1 teaspoon olive oil
4 (4-ounce) lamb chops,
   trimmed of all fat
Salt and freshly ground black
   pepper to taste
1 cup cubed button mushrooms
1 small onion, thinly sliced
1 small carrot, thinly sliced

1 small zucchini, thinly sliced
1 rib celery, thinly sliced
1 cup chicken stock
1 sprig fresh thyme
2 tablespoons chopped fresh
   parsley

Serves 4
Carb Level: Low

Per serving:	
Carbohydrate:	8.9 g
Protein:	20.7 g

A colorful and delicious blend of spring vegetables is the perfect pairing with these tender chops.

❧

1. Heat the oil in a large nonstick sauté pan over medium heat. Season the lamb chops with salt and pepper. Cook the lamb chops for about 2 minutes on each side or until brown. Transfer to a warm plate and keep warm.
2. Return the pan to medium heat and add the mushrooms, onion, carrot, zucchini, and celery. Cook, stirring frequently, for about 7 minutes or until tender. Add the stock, thyme, and parsley. Raise the heat to medium-high and bring to a boil. Reduce the heat to medium and simmer, covered, for 7 minutes. Add the reserved chops and simmer for an additional 3 minutes.
3. Serve on warm plates and spoon the vegetables and the sauce over the chops.

Weekend Guest Tip

Many weekend guests are early risers. As a courtesy, prepare your coffee pot the evening before so your guests just plug it in. It is also a nice touch to leave out coffee mugs and sugar/sugar substitute for easy access. Don't forget to have fresh milk or cream in the refrigerator.

Roast Pheasant with Cabbage

2 (3-pound) pheasants, trimmed of all fat and excess skin
Salt and freshly ground black pepper to taste
2 tablespoons olive oil
2 shallots, sliced
1 cup celery, chopped

1½ cups chicken stock
2 tablespoons brandy
1 head red cabbage, cored and shredded
1 tablespoon butter

1. Preheat the oven to 450°.
2. Wash the pheasants inside and out. Pat them dry and season with salt and pepper inside and out.
3. Heat the oil in a large roasting pan over medium-high heat on the stove. Add the pheasants breast side down. Cook for about 4 minutes or until golden brown. Continue to do this on all sides of the pheasant. Transfer the pheasants to the oven, breast side up, and roast for 15 minutes.
4. Add the shallots and the celery to the pheasants. Reduce the oven temperature to 375°. Roast for about 45 minutes or until the inside of the breast registers 170°. (Use an instant-read thermometer to take the internal temperature.) Transfer the pheasants to a warm platter and cover with foil to keep warm.
5. Bring a large pot of salted water to a boil.
6. Drain the liquid from the roasting pan through a fine-mesh sieve into a medium-size bowl. Skim off any fat that comes to the top of the liquid. Discard the vegetables.

(recipe continues on the next page)

Roast Pheasant with Cabbage (continued)

7. Place the roasting pan over high heat on the stove and add the stock and brandy. Bring to a boil, scraping up any browned bits from the bottom of the pan. Reduce the heat to medium and simmer for about 5 minutes. Strain through a fine-mesh sieve into a clean saucepan. Add the reserved liquid from the roasting pan and bring to a simmer.

8. Add the cabbage to the boiling water. Cover and cook for about 4 minutes. Drain the cabbage well and shake off any excess water. Return the cabbage to the pot and add the butter. Season with salt and pepper; mix well to combine.

9. Slice the breasts on an angle and remove the legs from the thighs on each bird. On warm plates, mound the cabbage on the bottom and arrange the sliced breasts, legs, and thighs on top of the cabbage. Drizzle the sauce over the pheasant.

Grilled Red Snapper with Basil Aioli

Vegetable oil, for oiling
4 (6-ounce) red snapper fillets
Salt and freshly ground black pepper to taste
¼ cup chopped fresh parsley
¼ cup chopped fresh basil
1 tablespoon mayonnaise
3 tablespoons olive oil
¼ cup chili sauce

Serves 4
Carb Level: Low

Per serving:	
Carbohydrate:	0.5 g
Protein:	4.9 g

If snapper isn't available, you can substitute salmon.

❧

1. Prepare a charcoal grill or preheat a gas grill to high heat. Make sure the grill grate is clean and lightly oiled to prevent sticking.

2. Season each fillet with salt and pepper. In a food processor or blender, combine the parsley, basil, mayonnaise, and olive oil; blend until smooth. Brush each fillet with the basil aioli.

3. Place the brushed fillets on the grill. Grill on each side for about 4 minutes or until done. Serve immediately with the chili sauce on the side.

White Wine–Poached Salmon

4 (6-ounce) portions of fresh Atlantic salmon, center-cut fillets, bones and skin removed

Salt and freshly ground black pepper to taste

¼ cup dry white wine

2 bay leaves

2 tablespoons chopped fresh dill

2 tablespoons lemon juice

1 tablespoon extra-virgin olive oil

1 tablespoon nonfat plain yogurt

2 medium cucumbers, peeled and halved lengthwise, seeded and cut into ¼-inch slices

4 sprigs fresh dill

1. Season the fillets with salt and pepper. Place the fish in a nonstick sauté pan large enough to hold the fillets. Add the wine, bay leaves, chopped dill, and enough water to come ⅛ inch up the side of the fish. Cover with a lid. Bring to a simmer and poach over medium heat for about 5 minutes. Turn off the heat and allow the fish to finish cooking, covered, for 6 minutes. Using a slotted spatula, gently remove the fillets from the pan to a warm plate; keep warm.

2. Whisk together the lemon juice and olive oil in a small bowl. Add the yogurt and cucumbers; toss well to combine. Season to taste with salt and pepper. Place the salmon fillets on a warm plate and spoon the cucumber garnish on top of each fillet. Garnish with fresh dill sprigs.

Chutney-Glazed Smoked Ham

*7-pound fully cooked bone-in
  ham*
½ cup peach or mango chutney
3 tablespoons Dijon mustard

½ teaspoon ground ginger
Rosemary sprigs for garnish

1. Preheat the oven to 325°.
2. Remove the skin and all but ¼ inch of the fat from the ham. Score the fat into 1-inch diamonds. Place the ham on a rack in a medium-size roasting pan. Roast the ham, uncovered, for 1½ hours.
3. Mix the chutney, mustard, and ginger in a small bowl. Brush this glaze all over the ham. Bake the ham for another 30 minutes or until the internal temperature registers 140°. Transfer the ham to a warm platter and brush with any remaining glaze. Allow the ham to rest for about 15 minutes. Slice and serve garnished with rosemary sprigs.

Serves 12
Carb Level: Low

Per serving:

Carbohydrate:	9.4 g
Protein:	0.3 g

You can use a spiral cut ham for this recipe to make the slicing step easier.

❧

Pesto-Baked Chicken

Serves 4
Carb Level: Low

Per serving:

Carbohydrate:	2.6 g
Protein:	36.2 g

Double or triple this recipe as needed for a group dinner or buffet luncheon.

∾

4 medium boneless, skinless
   chicken breast halves
1 tablespoon olive oil
2 cups finely chopped zucchini
   and/or yellow summer
   squash

2 tablespoons prepared pesto
2 tablespoons finely shredded
   Parmesan cheese or Asiago
   cheese

Rinse the chicken under cold running water and pat dry with paper towels. Heat the oil in a large nonstick sauté pan over medium heat. Cook the chicken, breast side down, for 4 minutes or until golden brown. Turn the chicken and add the squash. Cook, stirring the squash, for about 5 minutes or until the chicken is cooked through and the squash is tender. Transfer to warm plates and spoon the pesto over the breasts. Sprinkle with the grated cheese.

Making Your Own Pesto

You can prepare your own pesto by blending 1 cup fresh basil leaves, washed, dried, and stemmed; ¼ cup grated Parmesan cheese; 2 tablespoons toasted pine nuts; and approximately ¼ cup extra-virgin olive oil in a food processor until smooth. Add more oil as needed to adjust consistency, and season with salt and freshly ground black pepper.

Pork Roast

4 pound loin of pork, bone in
2 tablespoons extra-virgin
  olive oil
4 garlic cloves, sliced
2 sprigs fresh rosemary
1 bay leaf

1 cup dry white wine
Salt and freshly ground black
  pepper to taste

Serves 6
Carb Level: Low

Per serving:	
Carbohydrate:	1.5 g
Protein:	39.1 g

The pork will continue to cook after you remove it from the oven, adding an additional 5 to 8 degrees to the internal temperature.

1. Place the pork roast in a large plastic bag with a seal. Mix the oil, garlic, rosemary, bay leaf, wine, and salt and pepper in a small bowl until combined, then add to the pork. Massage the bag to ensure the pork is evenly coated with the marinade. Marinate for several hours in the refrigerator, turning occasionally.
2. Preheat oven to 450°.
3. Place the loin in a roasting pan set on a rack. Season with more salt and pepper and baste it with the marinade. Roast for about 20 minutes or until browned. Turn the heat down to 300° and roast for another 45 minutes to 1 hour or until the internal temperature is 150°. Baste with the pan liquids while roasting.
4. Allow the pork to rest for at least 15 minutes before slicing. Serve slices on warm plates.

Roasted Vidalia Onions

Serves 8
Carb Level: Low

Per serving:

Carbohydrate:	6.2 g
Protein:	0.8 g

Goes great with any grilled meat or fish.

4 Vidalia or other sweet onions, peeled and cut in half crosswise
3 tablespoons olive oil
2 tablespoons balsamic vinegar

Salt and freshly ground black pepper to taste
2 strips bacon, cut into 8 pieces

1. Prepare a charcoal grill or preheat a gas grill to high. Make sure the grill grate is clean and lightly oiled to prevent sticking.
2. Place each onion half, cut-side up, in a 10-inch square of foil. Drizzle the onions with the oil, vinegar, and season with salt and pepper. Turn the onions cut-side down. Place a piece of bacon on top of each onion. Fold the foil into packets.
3. Grill the onions for about 25 minutes or until they are tender and slightly charred. Allow the onions to cool in their packets for 15 minutes.
4. Remove the onions, discarding the bacon but reserving the juices. Serve warm or at room temperature and drizzle the juices over the top.

Balsamic Vinegar

This is a prized Italian specialty. Balsamic is manufactured from white Trebbiano grape juice. The rich burgundy color and sweetness are developed during an aging process in barrels of different woods in graduating sizes. Aged balsamic can be as expensive as a fine wine and well worth the investment. You need only a small amount of a quality balsamic to add punch to a dressing or sauce. If your balsamic is not the best quality, you can develop the flavor by bringing it to a low boil and allowing it to simmer until reduced by ¼ to ⅓; the concentration will improve the flavors.

Pork Crown Roast

8–9 pound crown roast of
   pork
5½ tablespoons olive oil,
   divided
Salt and freshly ground black
   pepper
Grated zest of 1 orange
4 large cloves garlic, minced
2 tablespoons chopped fresh
   rosemary

¾ cup dry white wine
½ cup fresh apple cider
1 cup chicken stock
1 tablespoon unsalted butter,
   at room temperature
2 tablespoons all-purpose flour

Serves 12–14
Carb Level: Low

Per serving:	
Carbohydrate:	2.3 g
Protein:	43.7 g

This is the perfect centerpiece for a large family get-together.

❧

1. Preheat oven to 425°.
2. Brush the roast with 4 tablespoons of olive oil and season well with salt and pepper. In a small bowl, mix together the orange zest, garlic, rosemary, and the remaining oil. Spread this mixture evenly over the meat, inside and out. Place the roast on a rack in a large roasting pan. Roast for 15 minutes and reduce the heat to 375°. Continue roasting for 45 minutes, rotating the roasting pan to ensure even cooking. Cook until the roast is browned and the internal temperature reads 150°, about 1½ hours.
3. Remove the roast from the oven and place on a cutting board. Tent with tin foil and allow to rest for at least 20 minutes. Deglaze the roasting pan over medium heat by adding the white wine and scraping the bottom of the pan to loosen any browned bits; stir to incorporate them into the wine. Simmer until the wine reduces by half. Add the apple cider and the stock. Season with salt and pepper and return the liquid to a boil.
4. In a small bowl, combine the butter with the flour; mix until well combined. Add this to the roasting pan, whisking, until the sauce has thickened, about 5 minutes. Strain through a fine-mesh sieve into a bowl. Remove any fat that accumulates at the top. Carve the roast at the table and pass the sauce around.

Cod Cakes

Serves 4
Carb Level: Low

Per serving:	
Carbohydrate:	9.7 g
Protein:	28.3 g

Serve the cakes with an Asian sauce or vinaigrette instead of tartar sauce and a side of stir-fried vegetables for a totally different variation.

1¼ pounds cod, cleaned and boned
4 scallions, chopped (about ⅓ cup)
2 tablespoons finely chopped fresh tarragon
1 egg, lightly beaten
3 dashes (or to taste) Tabasco sauce
Salt and freshly ground black pepper to taste
⅓ cup bread crumbs
3 tablespoons olive oil, divided
Tartar sauce for garnish

1. Cut the fish into large chunks and pulse in a food processor until coarsely chopped, or chop by hand using a very sharp knife. Transfer to a medium-size bowl and add the scallions, tarragon, egg, and Tabasco; mix well. Season with salt and pepper, then form 8 equal patties. Dredge them in the breadcrumbs and shake off any excess.
2. Heat 1 tablespoon of oil in a large nonstick sauté pan over medium-low heat. Cook the patties on each side for about 4 minutes or until they are golden brown. Turn them over and cook for about 5 minutes or until brown and cooked all the way through; add more oil as needed. Transfer to a warm plate and serve with tartar sauce on the side.

Snacks for Weekend Guests

When entertaining weekend guests, prepare a simple fruit platter and cheese and salami tray and leave it in the refrigerator for your guests to nibble on at their leisure.

Grilled Mushrooms and Peppers

1 cup olive oil
½ cup balsamic vinegar
Salt and freshly ground black
   pepper to taste
12 large portobello mushrooms,
   stems removed

6 large red, yellow, or green
   bell peppers, halved lengthwise, stemmed and seeded
Mixed salad greens

Serves 16	
Carb Level: Low	
Per serving:	
Carbohydrate:	6.1 g
Protein:	2.0 g

Easy to prepare in advance. Add your favorite grilled sausages and you have a delicious grilled entrée.

1. Prepare a charcoal grill or preheat a gas grill to high heat. Make sure the grill grate is clean and lightly oiled to prevent sticking.
2. In a medium-size bowl, whisk together the oil and vinegar, and season with salt and pepper. Brush the mushrooms and peppers with some of the dressing. Grill the mushrooms and peppers on each side until tender and slightly charred. Transfer to a large bowl and allow to cool for about 15 minutes.
3. Cut the mushroom and peppers into ½-inch-wide strips and return to the bowl. Mix in the remaining dressing and season with salt and pepper. Serve on a bed of mixed salad greens.

Coriander-Crusted Flank Steak

Serves 4
Carb Level: Low

Per serving:

Carbohydrate:	3.3 g
Protein:	33.8 g

The cilantro seasoning makes this a perfect pairing with either Mexican or Asian sides.

∾

2 tablespoons fresh-squeezed lemon juice
2 tablespoons soy sauce
2 tablespoons olive oil
2 tablespoons ground coriander
2 cloves garlic, minced
1½-pound beef flank steak, trimmed
¼ cup red wine
1 tablespoon black pepper
2 tablespoons chopped fresh cilantro
Fresh cilantro sprigs

1. Combine the lemon juice, soy sauce, oil, coriander, and garlic in a large plastic bag with a seal. Squeeze the bag to mix the marinade ingredients. Add the steak and squeeze the bag to ensure meat is evenly coated on both sides. Cover and refrigerate overnight, turning occasionally.
2. Prepare a charcoal grill or preheat a gas grill to high heat. Make sure the grill grate is clean and lightly oiled to prevent sticking
3. Remove the steak from the marinade. Transfer the marinade to a small saucepan and add the red wine. Season the steaks with pepper on both sides. Grill the steaks on each side for about 5 to 6 minutes or to the desired doneness. Transfer the meat to a platter and tent with tin foil; allow to rest for about 15 minutes.
4. Heat the marinade to a boil and then reduce heat to a simmer and cook until the sauce is slightly reduced. Strain the sauce through a fine-mesh sieve into a bowl. Slice the steak thinly across the grain and arrange on a platter. Drizzle the sauce over the steak. Sprinkle with chopped cilantro and garnish with cilantro sprigs.

Boneless Chicken Thighs with Major Grey's Chutney

6 boneless chicken thighs
Salt and freshly ground black
    pepper to taste
½ cup Major Grey's chutney

6 ounces goat cheese
2 tablespoons olive oil

Serves 6
Carb Level: Low

Per serving:	
Carbohydrate:	7.8 g
Protein:	30.3 g

Major Grey's is a traditional Indian-style chutney that can be found in Indian specialty stores.

∾

1. Loosen the skin on the chicken thighs. Season with salt and pepper. Evenly divide the chutney among the thighs; press the relish onto the thighs, under the skin. Press the goat cheese over the relish, evenly dividing it among the thighs. Stretch the skin over the stuffing and secure with a toothpick.
2. Preheat the oven to 375°.
3. Heat the oil in a large oven proof sauté pan over medium-high heat. Add the chicken thighs to the pan, skin side down, for about 5 minutes or until the skin is golden brown and crispy. Turn the thighs over and place the pan in the oven for about 20 to 25 minutes or until done.

Food Safety on the Web

A great up-to-date Web site is www.FoodSafety.gov for the latest information and technical details on foods and proper preparation.

Sautéed Ham
with a Cider Reduction

Serves 2
Carb Level: Moderate

Per serving:	
Carbohydrate:	16.3 g
Protein:	46.3 g

Try different fully cooked ham steaks from the meat counter of your supermarket to find the flavor you prefer.

∾

1½ cups apple cider
3 tablespoons cider vinegar
1 teaspoon mustard seeds
1 teaspoon Dijon mustard
1 tablespoon olive oil
1 pound fully cooked bone-in ham steak (about ½-inch thick)

1 small onion, finely chopped
2 tablespoons butter
1 tablespoon minced fresh flat-leaf parsley

1. In a small bowl, mix together the cider, vinegar, mustard seeds, and mustard.
2. Heat the oil in a large sauté pan over high heat and sauté the ham until it is golden and heated through, about 4 minutes on each side. Transfer the ham to a platter and keep warm.
3. In the same sauté pan, cook the onions over medium heat until golden. Stir in the cider mixture. Simmer, uncovered, for about 5 minutes or until slightly thickened. Add the butter and parsley to the sauce, and mix well. Pour the sauce over the ham and serve.

Barbecued Beef

1 slice bacon, cut into 1-inch
   pieces
½ cup chopped onion
½ cup ketchup
⅓ cup apple cider vinegar
1 teaspoon Dijon mustard
Dash of liquid smoke
1 teaspoon Worcestershire
   sauce
⅛ teaspoon salt

⅛ teaspoon freshly ground
   black pepper
4–8 packets sugar substitute
12 ounces roast beef, thinly
   sliced

Serves 4	
Carb Level: Moderate	
Per serving:	
Carbohydrate:	15.2 g
Protein:	14.7 g

This is a great way to
use leftover roast
beef or roast pork.

∾

1. In a medium-size saucepan over medium heat, cook the bacon until it just starts to crisp. Add the onion and cook for about 3 minutes, stirring, or until the bacon is crispy and the onion is tender.
2. Add the ketchup, apple cider vinegar, mustard, liquid smoke, Worcestershire sauce, salt, and pepper to the bacon mixture. Reduce the heat and simmer for about 15 minutes. Stir in 4 packets of the sugar substitute; add more substitute and adjust seasoning to taste. Add the sliced roast beef and simmer for 10 minutes.

Sautéed Swordfish in a White Wine Sauce

Serves 4
Carb Level: Moderate
Per serving:
Carbohydrate: 12.2 g
Protein: 38.5 g

If swordfish is not available, you can substitute snapper or halibut and reduce the cooking time accordingly.

∾

4 (7-ounce) swordfish steaks (about 1-inch thick)
Salt and freshly ground white pepper to taste
2 tablespoons canola oil
¼ cup dry white wine
2 tablespoons fresh-squeezed lemon juice
½ cup unsalted butter
1 tablespoon freshly chopped parsley leaves

5 scallions, finely sliced on the bias, white parts only
1 tablespoon capers, drained and rinsed
1 large ripe tomato, peeled, seeded, and cut into ¼-inch dice

1. Season the swordfish with salt and pepper on both sides. Heat the oil in a large sauté pan over medium-high heat. Cook the fish on 1 side for about 6 minutes or until lightly browned. Turn the fillet over, reduce the heat to medium, and cook for about 4 more minutes or until browned. Cover and cook until the fish is done, about 5 minutes. To check for doneness, insert a thin-bladed knife in the thickest part of the fish. The flesh should be flaky and no translucence should be apparent. Transfer the fish to a platter and cover to keep warm.

2. Pour off any oil remaining in the pan and add the wine and lemon juice. Raise the heat to high and scrape the bottom of the pan to loosen any browned bits. Simmer until the sauce reduces by half. Stir in the butter 1 piece at a time. Add the parsley, scallions, capers, tomato, and season with salt and pepper. Pour the sauce over the fish and serve immediately.

Grilled Mediterranean Grouper

Vinaigrette:

1 cup extra-virgin olive oil
2 tablespoons tarragon vinegar
1/2 cup tomatoes, peeled, seeded, and diced
1/3 cup pitted and halved kalamata olives
1 medium shallot, thinly sliced
1/2 teaspoon minced garlic
Salt and freshly ground black pepper to taste

Fennel:

2 medium fennel bulbs, trimmed
2 tablespoons extra-virgin olive oil
Salt and freshly ground white pepper to taste

Grouper:

4 (6-ounce) grouper fillets
2 tablespoons vegetable oil
Salt and freshly ground white pepper to taste
2 tablespoons minced fresh chives for garnish

Serves 4
Carb Level: Low

Per serving:

Carbohydrate:	10.0 g
Protein:	15.9 g

You can substitute salmon if fresh grouper is not available.

∾

1. To prepare the vinaigrette: Combine the olive oil, vinegar, tomatoes, olives, shallot, garlic, and salt and pepper in a medium-size bowl; set aside.
2. Prepare a charcoal grill or preheat a gas grill over medium-high heat. Make sure the grill grate is clean and lightly oiled to prevent sticking.
3. To prepare the fennel: Cut the fennel bulbs in half lengthwise. Slice each half lengthwise into 1/4-inch-thick slices. Try to keep each slice attached at the root end. Brush the fennel with olive oil and season with salt and pepper.
4. Grill the fennel for about 5 minutes on each side until tender and slightly charred; set aside and keep warm.
5. To prepare the grouper: Clean and lightly oil the grill.
6. Brush the fillets with the oil and season with salt and pepper. Grill the fish for about 4 minutes on 1 side, then turn the fillet and cook for an additional 2 minutes or until done. To check for doneness, insert a thin-bladed knife in the thickest part of the fish. The flesh should be flaky and no translucence should be apparent.
7. Serve the fennel under the fish and spoon the vinaigrette over the fish. Garnish with fresh chives and serve immediately.

Cauliflower Vichyssoise

Serves 4

Carb Level: Moderate

Per serving:

Carbohydrate:	14.2 g
Protein:	2.7 g

This satisfying soup can be served hot or cold.

&

1 tablespoon vegetable oil
2 medium leeks, white parts only, sliced
1 medium onion, diced
1 large head cauliflower, cut into florets
4 cups chicken stock

Salt and freshly ground white pepper to taste
¼ cup extra-virgin olive oil
1 tablespoon finely minced chives for garnish

1. Heat the oil in a large soup pot over medium heat. Cook the leeks and onion for 3 to 4 minutes, stirring, until tender. Be careful not to overcook the leeks and onion; they should retain their original color.
2. Add the cauliflower and stock and bring to a boil. Reduce the heat and simmer, covered, for about 20 minutes or until the cauliflower is tender.
3. Transfer the soup to a blender and purée until smooth. Return the soup to the pot to warm; season with salt and pepper.
4. Serve the soup in warm soup bowls and garnish with a drizzle of extra-virgin olive oil and a sprinkling of fresh chives.

Are You Losing Vitamins?

Vitamins are destroyed by heat, water, air, and fat. Different cooking methods will dictate the amount of vitamins retained or lost. For example, Vitamin C is an oxygen-sensitive and water-soluble vitamin. Cooking 1 cup of cabbage in 4 cups of water loses 90 percent of the natural vitamin C. Cooking 4 cups of cabbage in 1 cup of water retains about 50 percent of the natural vitamin C.

Beef Tenderloin with Belgian Endive

1½ teaspoons butter, divided
2½ teaspoons canola oil, divided
8 Belgian endives, washed, cored,
    and cut in half lengthwise
Salt and freshly ground black
    pepper to taste
2 shallots, minced
½ cup dry white wine

1 cup veal or chicken stock
4 (5-ounce) beef tenderloin fillets
2 cups button mushrooms, sliced
1 clove garlic, minced
2 tablespoons chopped fresh
    flat-leaf parsley

Serves 4
Carb Level: Moderate

Per serving:	
Carbohydrate:	17.3 g
Protein:	26.2 g

The endives add a nice change of pace to a traditional fillet dinner with mushrooms.

∾

1. Heat 1 teaspoon of the butter and 1 teaspoon of the oil in a large nonstick sauté pan over medium-low heat. Add the endives to the pan in a single layer. Season with salt and pepper. Cook, covered, for 15 minutes. Turn them over, cover, and cook for another 10 minutes. Transfer the endives to a plate and keep warm.

2. In the same sauté pan, add the shallots and the remaining ½ teaspoon of butter, and increase the heat to medium. Cook for about 4 minutes or until the shallots are softened. Add the wine and bring it to a boil for 5 minutes or until the wine is reduced by half. Add the stock and bring to a boil. Reduce to a simmer and cook until the liquid is reduced by ⅓. Season with salt and pepper. Remove from the heat and keep warm.

3. Season the beef with salt and pepper. Heat the remaining oil in a medium sauté pan over high heat. Add the beef and cook for about 3 minutes or until brown. Brown the other side. (The beef should be medium-rare at this point; cook longer if preferred.) Transfer the meat to a plate and keep warm.

5. Return the pan to medium heat. Add the mushrooms and season with salt and pepper. Cook for about 5 minutes or until the mushrooms are tender. Add the garlic and sauté for 30 seconds more. Toss in the parsley and stir to mix.

6. Place each tenderloin in the center of a warm dinner plate. Arrange the endive around each tenderloin. Spoon the sauce over the beef and then top with the mushrooms.

Fish Stew

Serves 4

Carb Level: Moderate

Per serving:

Carbohydrate:	20.0 g
Protein:	42.8 g

Fish stock can be purchased at any specialty food store.

12 ounces bass or grouper fillets
12 ounces medium shrimp,
   peeled and deveined
8 ounces fresh mussels
1½ fennel bulbs
1 tablespoon olive oil
1 medium onion, thinly sliced
2 medium leeks, thinly sliced
3 cloves garlic, minced

6 cups fish stock
4 very ripe plum tomatoes, peeled,
   seeded, cored, and chopped
2 sprigs fresh thyme
2 pinches of saffron threads
Salt and freshly ground black
   pepper to taste
1 tablespoon chopped fresh
   tarragon for garnish

1. Cut the fish into medium-size chunks and place in a bowl. Add the shrimp and refrigerate.

2. Wash the mussels very well in a few changes of cold water. Scrub off any grit stuck to the mussels and remove the beards. (Your fish purveyor will clean the mussels if you ask.) Place the mussels in a medium-size saucepan and add enough cold water to cover by about 1 inch. Bring to a boil, covered, over medium-high heat. Steam the mussels until they open. Discard any that remain closed. Remove the mussels from the pan and lift the meat from the shells; discard the shells. Return the mussels to the saucepan. Reserve the flavorful cooking liquid.

3. To prepare the fennel, remove any discolored outer layers from the bulb. Trim the root end and trim off the feathery top. Cut the bulb in half lengthwise and then cut crosswise into very thin slices.

4. Heat the oil in a large saucepan over medium heat. Add the fennel, onions, and leeks. Cook slowly, uncovered and stirring often, for about 8 minutes or until tender. Stir in the garlic and cook for another 2 to 3 minutes until soft. Add the fish stock, tomatoes, thyme, and saffron. Season with salt and pepper. Cover and simmer for about 10 minutes.

5. Add the fish and shrimp to the stew. Cover and cook over medium heat for about 8 minutes or until the fish and shrimp are cooked. Add the mussels with their cooking liquid to the stew. Adjust seasoning to taste.

6. Ladle the stew into warm soup bowls with equal amounts of fish in each. Garnish with chopped tarragon.

Venison Medallions with Cranberry Dijon Chutney

1 cup fresh cranberries
1 teaspoon honey
1 tablespoon Dijon mustard
2 teaspoons butter, divided
Salt and freshly ground black
    pepper to taste
8 (2-$\frac{1}{2}$ ounce) venison
    medallions
2 small shallots, minced
2 cups quartered domestic
    mushrooms
1 cup dry red wine
$\frac{1}{4}$ cup cider vinegar
$\frac{1}{2}$ cup chicken stock
1 tablespoon red currant jelly

Serves 4	
Carb Level: Moderate	
Per serving:	
Carbohydrate:	14.1 g
Protein:	24.7 g

Venison should never be cooked past medium or it will become very dry and tough.

1. In a small nonstick sauté pan, combine the cranberries, honey, mustard, and 1 teaspoon of the butter. Season with salt and pepper. Cook over low heat for about 3 to 5 minutes until the cranberries just start to pop. Remove from the heat and set aside.
2. Season the venison with salt and pepper. Melt the remaining butter in a large nonstick sauté pan over high heat until very hot. Add the venison and sear for about 2 minutes or until golden brown. Turn over and sear for another 2 minutes. The meat should be medium-rare at this point. Transfer to a warm platter and keep warm.
3. Return the sauté pan to medium heat. Add the shallots and cook for about 2 minutes or until tender. Stir in the mushrooms and cook until softened. Add the wine, the stock, and the vinegar, and scrape the bottom of the pan with a wooden spoon to loosen any browned bits. Raise the heat to high and cook for about 10 minutes or until the liquid is reduced to about $\frac{1}{2}$ cup. Stir in the jelly and adjust seasoning to taste.
4. Spoon a small amount of the cranberry sauce on top of each venison medallion. Ladle the sauce on top and around the venison.

Roasted Eggplant Napoleon with Marinated Goat Cheese

Serves 6
Carb Level: Moderate

Per serving:

Carbohydrate:	12.7 g
Protein:	9.0 g

An attractive and flavorful starter course. Everything can be prepared beforehand and assembled just before serving.

~

2 cloves garlic, minced
1 tablespoon fresh thyme
   leaves
3 teaspoons olive oil, divided
4 ounces fresh goat cheese
1 large eggplant
Salt and freshly ground black
   pepper to taste
10 ounces fresh spinach,
   washed and stems removed
2 small red bell peppers,
   roasted, peeled, seeded,
   and diced

3 very ripe plum tomatoes,
   peeled, seeded, cored,
   and diced
3 tablespoons coarsely
   chopped fresh basil
Juice of 1 lemon

1. Mix half of the minced garlic, thyme, black pepper, and 1 teaspoon of the oil in a large bowl. Crumble the goat cheese into the bowl, and lightly toss to ensure the cheese is evenly coated with the marinade. Cover and allow to sit at room temperature.

2. Trim off the stem ends from the eggplant. Cut the eggplant crosswise into $1/8$-inch slices. Lay the slices on a baking sheet and sprinkle them with salt. Allow them to sit for about 10 minutes. The salt will help extract some of the bitterness from the eggplant.

3. Preheat the oven to 450°.

4. Using a paper towel, blot away the liquid released from the eggplant and brush off the salt. Pat the skin very dry. Brush both sides of the eggplant with the remaining oil. Roast for about 5 minutes or until the slices begin to slightly color. Remove from the oven.

(recipe continues on the next page)

Roasted Eggplant Napoleon
with Marinated Goat Cheese (continued)

5. Heat the remaining oil in a large nonstick sauté pan over medium heat. Add the remaining minced garlic and cook for about 1 minute or until it just starts to color. Add the spinach to the pan and season with salt and pepper. Cover and cook over medium heat for about 2 minutes, until all of the spinach has wilted. Remove from the heat and drain off the excess water. Mix the spinach with the red peppers in a medium-size bowl.

6. Mix the tomatoes, basil, and lemon juice, and salt and pepper in a small bowl.

7. To assemble, place a slice of the eggplant on each serving plate, spoon the spinach and pepper mixture in the center of the eggplant, and top with another layer of eggplant; add the marinated goat cheese for the next layer, and top with the tomato vinaigrette.

Fried Green Tomatoes

1 cup extra-virgin olive oil
2 large or 3 small green
  tomatoes
Yellow cornmeal, for dredging

Salt and freshly ground black
  pepper to taste

1. Heat the oil in a medium-size sauté pan over medium heat.
2. Cut the tomatoes into ¼-inch slices. Season both sides with salt and pepper. Dredge them in cornmeal, coating well on both sides.
3. Fry them in the oil until golden brown, turning them only once. Drain them of excess oil on paper towels. Serve immediately.

Serves 4
Carb Level: Moderate

Per serving:	
Carbohydrate:	18.1 g
Protein:	2.6 g

This is a great accompaniment to an end-of-summer BBQ dinner or lunch.

Baked Cod with Tomatoes, Capers, and Sautéed Spinach

Serves 4

Carb Level: Moderate

Per serving:

Carbohydrate:	14.3 g
Protein:	46.2 g

You can substitute any firm fish for the cod, such as grouper or haddock.

❧

1 teaspoon butter, divided
2 teaspoons olive oil, divided
2 large very ripe tomatoes, peeled, seeded, cored, and diced
1 cup fish stock
3 tablespoons capers, well drained
Salt and freshly ground black pepper to taste

⅓ cup fresh bread crumbs
1 tablespoon chopped fresh chives
1 tablespoon chopped fresh flat-leaf parsley
4 (5-ounce) cod fillets
1 pound fresh spinach, washed and stems removed

1. Preheat the oven to 450°. Using ½ teaspoon of the butter, lightly coat a casserole dish large enough to hold the fish in a single layer.
2. Heat 1 teaspoon of oil in a medium sauté pan over medium-high heat. Add the tomatoes and cook for about 2 minutes. Add the stock and capers; bring to a boil. Reduce the heat to low and simmer for about 10 minutes. Season with salt and pepper and cover to keep warm.
3. In a small bowl, combine the bread crumbs, chives, parsley, and the remaining oil; mix well.
4. Season the cod on both sides with salt and pepper. Lay the fillets in the buttered casserole. Top each fillet with an equal amount of the bread crumb mixture. Bake for about 8 minutes or until the cod is almost done. Turn the broiler on and broil the fish for about 1 minute or until the tops are golden brown and the fish is done. To check the fish for doneness, insert a thin-bladed knife into the thickest part of the fish. The flesh should be white and flaky; no translucence should be apparent. Remove the fish from the broiler and keep warm.
5. Melt the remaining butter in a large nonstick sauté pan over high heat. Add the spinach to the pan and season with salt and pepper. Cover and cook for about 2 minutes or until the spinach has wilted.
6. Place a small pile of spinach in the center of a warm dinner plate. Place a cod fillet on top of the spinach and pour the sauce around the fish.

Artichoke, Cucumber, and Tomato Salad

2 English cucumbers, peeled
2 teaspoons lemon juice
1 tablespoon olive oil
Salt and freshly ground black
    pepper to taste
4 very ripe plum tomatoes,
    peeled, seeded, cored, and
    chopped

6 ounces mesclun salad,
    washed and dried
1 cup quartered canned arti-
    choke hearts, drained

Serves 4
Carb Level: Moderate

Per serving:	
Carbohydrate:	19.5 g
Protein:	5.3 g

This flavorful salad has a wonderful blend of textures and flavors. It goes great with grilled meats.

1. Split the cucumbers in half and use a spoon to scoop out the seeds. Slice the cucumbers into $1/8$-inch slices. Drain the cucumbers and pat dry. Transfer the cucumbers to a medium-size bowl.
2. In a small bowl, whisk together the lemon juice, olive oil, and salt and pepper; add the tomatoes and stir well to combine.
3. Add $1/4$ of the prepared vinaigrette to the cucumbers and toss well to coat.
4. Place the mesclun in a large bowl. Add the remaining vinaigrette and toss to coat. Place a mound of greens on a chilled plate and top with the marinated cucumbers. Arrange the artichokes around the plate.

Flowers on Your Food?

Spring and summer brunches are always more festive when decorated with fresh flowers and greens. The following common flowers are "food safe": Bee Balm, Calendula, Chamomile, Chives, Daylilies, Impatiens, Lilac, Nasturtiums, Pansies, Roses, Violets. Be careful not to use any flowers that have been exposed to pesticides.

Roasted Rabbit with Garlic

Serves 4
Carb Level: Low

Per serving:

Carbohydrate:	9.9 g
Protein:	24.7 g

Rabbits are available in the frozen foods section in many supermarkets. Thaw according to package directions.

16 large cloves garlic, unpeeled
1 teaspoon vegetable oil
2 (10-ounce) rabbit saddles, well tied with butcher's twine to form 2 small tight roasts
Salt and freshly ground black pepper to taste

½ cup dry white wine
½ cup chicken stock
½ cup water
1 teaspoon fresh thyme leaves
1 teaspoon Dijon mustard
½ teaspoon unsalted butter
½ teaspoon honey

1. Preheat the oven to 375°.
2. Place the garlic in a small saucepan and add cold water to cover by 1 inch. Bring to a simmer over medium-high heat and cook for about 5 minutes. Remove from the heat and drain well; set aside.
3. Heat the oil on medium in a large nonstick sauté pan large enough to hold the rabbit uncrowded in a single layer. Season the rabbit with salt and pepper and place in the hot pan. Brown all sides, add the unpeeled garlic, and place in the oven. Roast for about 15 minutes or until the internal temperature of the meat reads 160°. Remove the rabbit from the oven and transfer to a warm plate; cover to keep warm.
4. Place the sauté pan with the unpeeled garlic in it over medium heat. Stir in the wine, stock, water, and thyme. Increase the heat and bring to a boil. Reduce the heat to medium and simmer for about 6 minutes or until the liquid is reduced by half. Remove the garlic cloves from the pan with a slotted spoon and set aside. Strain the sauce through a fine-mesh sieve into a small saucepan. Whisk in the mustard, butter, and honey and season with salt and pepper. Cover and keep warm.
5. Slice each rabbit saddle into 8 equal slices. Squeeze the roasted garlic cloves out of the skins. Arrange the garlic cloves around the rabbit and spoon the sauce on top.

Roasting Garlic
The roasted garlic cloves add an amazing complexity to this dish. They become much more mellow in flavor when they roast for a long period of time.

Roasted Grouper with Tomatoes

3 tablespoons olive oil
2 dried hot peppers
2 cloves garlic, peeled and
   lightly crushed
2 cups tomatoes (fresh or
   canned), peeled, seeded,
   and chopped
1 teaspoon dried rosemary
Salt and freshly ground black
   pepper to taste

1 large or 2 small grouper fillets, about 1 pound total
½ cup fresh parsley, minced
Freshly grated Parmesan cheese

Serves 4
Carb Level: Moderate

Per serving:	
Carbohydrate:	18.4 g
Protein:	16.9 g

Lightly stewing the
tomatoes enhances
the flavor of the sauce.

❧

1. Heat the oil in a large sauté pan over medium-high heat. Add the hot peppers and garlic, and cook, stirring, until the garlic is golden brown. Remove and discard the peppers and the garlic.

2. Add the tomatoes to the same pan and cook, stirring, until the tomatoes begin to liquefy. Add the rosemary, and salt and pepper; cook for about 5 minutes, then gently place the fillets in the pan. Cover the sauté pan and cook over medium heat for about 7 minutes or until the fish is done. To check for doneness, insert a thin-bladed knife into the thickest part of the fish. The flesh should be white, opaque, and flaky; no translucence should be apparent.

3. Carefully remove the fillets from the pan and set on a warm platter. Add some of the parsley to the sauce along with the cheese. Allow the cheese to melt. Spoon the sauce over the fish and garnish with the remaining chopped parsley.

Veal Saltimboca

<table>
<tr><td>Serves 2</td></tr>
</table>

Serves 2

Carb Level: Moderate

Per serving:

Carbohydrate:	17.1 g
Protein:	39.6 g

This recipe serves 2 as a starter course or 1 as an entrée.

∾

2 (2-ounce) veal cutlets
Salt and freshly ground black
   pepper to taste
2 fresh sage leaves, chopped
1 ounce mozzarella cheese,
   sliced
1 thin slice of prosciutto
2 large eggs, lightly beaten
   and seasoned with parsley,
   nutmeg, Parmesan cheese,
   salt and pepper
½ cup bread crumbs, sea-
   soned with salt, pepper,
   and Parmesan cheese
1 tablespoon butter

1 tablespoon extra-virgin
   olive oil
½ cup veal stock
¼ cup Marsala wine
¼ cup vermouth
1 tablespoon tomato paste
1 teaspoon finely chopped
   fresh parsley
1 sprig fresh parsley for
   garnish

1. Pound the veal between 2 sheets of plastic wrap with the flat side of a meat mallet to a uniform thickness of about ⅛ inch.
2. Lay the cutlets on a cutting board and season them with salt and pepper and the fresh sage. Lay a slice of mozzarella followed by a slice of prosciutto on the cutlet and top with the second veal cutlet. Seal the edges by pressing them together with your fingers.
3. Carefully dip the veal packet in the egg wash and then the bread crumbs. Press the bread crumbs firmly into the veal so that the packet stays together.
4. Heat the butter and oil in a medium-size sauté pan over medium heat. Cook the veal on both sides until golden brown and cooked through, about 7 minutes.

(recipe continues on the next page)

Veal Saltimboca (continued)

5. Combine the stock, Marsala, vermouth, tomato paste, salt and pepper, and parsley in a medium-size nonreactive saucepot. Bring to a boil, reduce the heat to low, and simmer until reduced by half.
6. Spoon some sauce on the bottom of a warm plate and lay the veal on top. Spoon a bit more sauce on top of the veal and garnish with the parsley sprig.

Making Veal Stock

Veal stock is a very flavorful broth made from simmering roasted veal bones, vegetables, and herbs together for 8 hours. The end result is a viscous and rich stock that can be used as a base for any sauce, soup, or braising liquid. Demi-glaze is when veal stock is reduced by half of its original volume. It is very intense in flavor and usually needs to be diluted with some water. You can buy this in specialty food stores.

Marinated Grilled Steak Strips

Serves 4
Carb Level: Low

Per serving:	
Carbohydrate:	1.4 g
Protein:	8.3 g

An outdoor grilling favorite. Serve with roasted assorted vegetables and a crispy salad for a summer night treat.

∾

4 (8-ounce) New York strip
  steaks, trimmed of all
  visible fat
Salt and freshly ground black
  pepper to taste
Fresh herbs for garnish

Marinade

³⁄₄ cup dry red wine
1 teaspoon minced garlic or
  2 cloves garlic, crushed
1 tablespoon dry sherry
¹⁄₂ teaspoon dried thyme,
¹⁄₂ teaspoon dried basil

1. For the marinade: Combine all the ingredients in a small saucepan. Simmer, uncovered, over medium heat for 15 minutes. Remove from heat and allow to cool to room temperature. Refrigerate in a sealed container until ready to use. Marinade can be prepared up to 48 hours in advance.
2. Place the steaks in a large plastic storage bag with a leak-proof seal. Pour the marinade over the steaks and squeeze out as much of the air as possible before sealing the bag. Refrigerate for at least 4 hours or up to 24 hours.
3. To grill: Preheat the grill. Lightly oil the grilling rack to ensure the steaks do not stick. Remove the steaks from the marinade, reserving the marinade for basting.
4. Season the steaks with salt and pepper. Grill, basting frequently with the marinade. For steaks of approximately 1¹⁄₂-inch thickness, grill 8 to 12 minutes per side for medium-rare. Increase the cooking time by 3 minutes per side for medium, 5 minutes for medium-well, and 7 minutes for well-done.
5. Transfer the steaks to a warmed platter and let the steaks rest for about 5 minutes before serving to allow the natural juices to reabsorb. Adjust seasoning to taste. Serve immediately, garnished with fresh herbs, if desired.

Grilled Swordfish with Olive Tapenade

8 (7-ounce) swordfish steaks
6 small leeks, washed well
Salt and freshly ground black
    pepper to taste
½ cup, plus 1 tablespoon
    extra-virgin olive oil, plus
    more for brushing
¼ cup pitted oil-cured olives
1 small clove garlic, peeled

1½ loosely packed cups
    arugula leaves
¼ cup fresh flat-leaf parsley
    leaves
¼ teaspoon dried oregano

Serves 8
Carb Level: Moderate

Per serving:

Carbohydrate:	15.5 g
Protein:	36.4 g

A great recipe for an evening barbecue with friends

❧

1. Prepare a charcoal grill or preheat a gas grill to high. Make sure the grill grate is clean and lightly oiled to prevent sticking.
2. Season the swordfish and the leeks with salt and pepper, and coat with 3 tablespoons of the oil. Allow the fish and leeks to marinate at room temperature for about 1 hour or until ready to grill.
3. To prepare the tapenade, combine the olives, garlic, arugula, parsley, oregano, and salt and pepper in a food processor. With the machine running, drizzle in the remaining oil. Add 1½ tablespoons of hot water, and purée until smooth.
4. Place the fish and the leeks on the grill. After cooking the leeks for 5 minutes, remove from the grill and flip the fish. Cook the fish for another 5 minutes until it is cooked through. Remove the fish from the grill and place on a plate. Arrange the leeks on a platter and place the fish on top of the leeks. Spoon the tapenade over the hot fish and serve immediately.

If You Don't Have Access to a Grill

If the weather ruins your outdoor grilling plans, use the broiler for this recipe. Broil the fish about 3 inches from the heat source and turn once. Finish cooking the fish in a preheated 375° oven if needed.

Pecan-Crusted Catfish with Wilted Greens

<table>
<tr><td>

Serves 8

Carb Level: Moderate

Per serving:

Carbohydrate:	17.2 g
Protein:	32.4 g

A crispy Southern-style method for fish preparation—add Southern-style greens to this dish for a perfect pairing.

∾

</td><td>

2 cups ground pecans
2 cups pecan pieces
½ cup all-purpose flour
Salt and freshly ground black
   pepper to taste
1 teaspoon cayenne pepper
1 large egg

3 tablespoons milk
8 (6-ounce) catfish or red
   snapper fillets

</td></tr>
</table>

1. Preheat oven to 450°.
2. Combine the pecans and spread out on a plate. Mix together the flour, salt and pepper, and cayenne. Spread this out on a plate. Whisk together the egg and the milk in a shallow bowl.
3. Coat each fillet with the flour, dip in the egg wash, then firmly press the pecans onto the fish, coating completely.
4. Arrange the fish on an oiled baking sheet in a single layer. Be careful not to overlap. Place in the oven and bake for about 15 minutes. To check for doneness, insert the tip of a thin-bladed knife into the thickest part of the fish. The flesh should be opaque and flaky. Serve immediately.

Cheese Platters Are Great for Parties

A nice selection of cheeses is a great addition to any get-together no matter how formal. Vary the intensity of flavors, and include a sheep milk cheese, a cow milk cheese, and a goat milk cheese. You can find these types of cheeses at any specialty food store. Serve the cheese at room temperature with nuts and marinated olives. You can also add a roasted vegetable spread and whole grain crackers. Garnish with fresh greens and serve on a nice wooden cheese board.

Roasted Salmon
with Goat Cheese and Tarragon

6 (7-ounce) salmon fillets,
  skin on

$\frac{1}{4}$ cup fresh-squeezed lemon
  juice

Salt and freshly ground black
  pepper to taste

2 cloves garlic, crushed

6 tablespoons olive oil

6 ounces soft, creamy goat
  cheese, at room temperature

3 tablespoons minced fresh
  tarragon, divided

3 tablespoons chopped fresh
  chives, divided

Serves 6
Carb Level: Low

Per serving:	
Carbohydrate:	2.0 g
Protein:	42.8 g

The tang of quality goat cheese is a perfect pairing with the rich flavor of roasted salmon.

1. Place the fish in a shallow baking dish in a single layer; do not overlap.
2. In a small bowl, whisk together the lemon juice, salt and pepper, garlic, and oil; pour over the fish. Cover and refrigerate for 2 hours, turning the fish several times.
3. Preheat oven to 450°.
4. Lay the marinated fish, skin side down, on a baking sheet lined with parchment paper. Bake the fish for about 10 minutes or until just done.
5. Meanwhile, beat the cheese with the back of a rubber spatula until soft and smooth. Mix with $1\frac{1}{2}$ tablespoons each of the tarragon and chives.
6. Remove the fillets from the oven and discard the skin. Transfer to a platter. Sprinkle a bit of salt and pepper on top of the fillets. Place a large dollop of the cheese mixture on top of each fillet. Garnish with the remaining herbs.

Mussels Steamed in White Wine

Serves 4

Carb Level: Moderate

Per serving:

Carbohydrate:	20.0 g
Protein:	37.3 g

This is one of the most traditional methods for preparing fresh mussels.

8 cups fresh mussels
1½ teaspoons olive oil
3 small shallots, minced
2 cloves garlic, minced
1½ cups dry white wine
2 bay leaves
4 very ripe tomatoes, peeled, seeded, cored, and chopped

Salt and freshly ground black pepper to taste
2 tablespoons chopped fresh flat-leaf parsley for garnish

1. Wash the mussels very well in 3 changes of clean water. Scrub off any grit and remove the beards. Discard any open mussels.
2. Heat the oil in a large sauté pan over medium-high heat. Add the shallots and cook for about 1 minute or until tender. Add the garlic and cook until it just starts to brown. Add the wine and the bay leaves, then stir in the mussels. Cover and cook for about 4 minutes or until the mussels open. Discard any that do not open. Remove the pan from the heat. Using a slotted spoon, transfer the mussels to shallow soup bowls. Strain the cooking liquid through a fine-mesh sieve into a medium-size saucepan.
3. Add the tomatoes to the saucepan and bring to a boil. Season with salt and pepper. Ladle the sauce over the mussels and garnish with chopped parsley. Serve immediately.

CHAPTER 15

Entertaining

Lemon Chicken Drumettes	256
Spanish Marinated Olives ❖	257
Smoked Shrimp with Horseradish Cream ❖	258
Hard-Boiled Eggs Stuffed with Mushrooms and Cheese	259
Mussel Salad with Green Beans	260
Mexican-Style Shrimp Cocktail ❖	261
Orange-Cucumber Salsa ❖	262
Stuffed Zucchini	263
Mushrooms Au Gratin ❖	264
Stewed Pepper and Tomato Purée ❖	265
Eggplant Topped with Gruyère Cheese ❖	266
Avocado and Tomato Dip ❖	267
Spicy Olive and Walnut Tapenade ❖	268
Crab Salad ❖	268
Green Beans with Shallots and Rosemary ❖	269
Chicken Pâté	270
Tuna Tapenade ❖	271
Shrimp Scampi ❖	271
Salmon Fillets with Basil ❖	272
Scallops in an Herbed Tomato Sauce	273
Beef with Cucumber	274
Chicken with Nectarine Salsa ❖	275
Sautéed Spinach with Pine Nuts ❖	276
Grilled Tomatoes ❖	277
Grilled Radicchio ❖	277

❖ Indicates Easy Recipe ❖

Lemon Chicken Drumettes

Serves 10

Carb Level: Low

Per serving:

Carbohydrate:	7.4 g
Protein:	20.0 g

Makes a tasty appetizer for any get together.

ᘐ

4 pounds chicken drumettes
Salt and freshly ground black
    pepper to taste
¼ cup orange juice
2 tablespoons grated fresh
    ginger
3 tablespoons vegetable oil
5 cloves garlic, finely chopped
1 cup very finely chopped
    fresh cilantro (about 3
    bunches)

1–2 fresh jalapeño peppers,
    seeded and very finely
    chopped
2 teaspoons ground cumin
1 teaspoon ground coriander
    seeds
Lemon wedges for garnish
    (optional)

1. Preheat oven to 500°. Line 2 baking sheets with aluminum foil.
2. Cut off the wing tips from the wings to make drumettes if necessary. Arrange the drumettes on the foil, trying not to overlap them. Season with salt and pepper. Place the baking pans on the top rack of the oven until brown, about 5 minutes. Turn the drumettes over and return to the oven to brown for another 3 minutes. Transfer the drumettes to paper towels and set aside, saving the pans.
3. Bring ¼ cup of water to a boil, then stir in the orange juice. Combine this mixture with the ginger and 1 cup of water in a blender or food processor; purée to a smooth consistency.
4. In a large heavy skillet, heat the oil over medium-high heat. Add the garlic and cook until softened, about 2 minutes (be careful not to burn the garlic; reduce the heat if necessary). Reduce the heat and stir in the cilantro, jalapeños, cumin, coriander, and about 1 teaspoon of salt. Add the orange-ginger mixture to the pan and stir to mix. Turn up the heat, bring to a boil, and reduce the liquid until the sauce is thick, like salsa. Adjust seasoning to taste.

(recipe continues on the next page)

Lemon Chicken Drumettes (continued)

5. To serve, arrange the drumettes on a serving platter and top with the warm sauce. Garnish with lemon wedges surrounding the drumettes.

Anatomy of a Chicken Wing

Chicken wings are separated into 3 joints. Drumettes are the top joint of the wing and are like miniature drumsticks. They may be purchased precut, or the whole wing may be separated at the joints. The wing tips can be discarded or used for chicken stock. The middle section may be also used for this recipe, but the drumettes are much easier to eat as an appetizer.

Spanish Marinated Olives

36 large good-quality green olives (held in a brine, but not a marinade), unpitted
½ teaspoon cracked peppercorns
1 teaspoon fresh thyme
1 sprig fresh rosemary
½ teaspoon dried oregano
3 bay leaves
4 cloves garlic, crushed
Finely grated zest from 1 lemon
¼ cup balsamic vinegar
About 1 cup extra-virgin olive oil to cover

Serves 12	
Carb Level: Low	
Per serving:	
Carbohydrate:	2.3 g
Protein:	0.6 g

These will keep in the refrigerator for up to 4 weeks.

Drain the olives. Place several at a time on a flat surface and crush them slightly with a large wide-blade chef's knife, without altering their shape. This opens them up just enough to marinate throughout. In a large bowl, toss together the olives with all the ingredients *except* the olive oil. Place them in a preserving jar or plastic container with tight-fitting lid and cover the olives with the olive oil. Marinate for a least 1 week in the refrigerator. Keep refrigerated, but return to room temperature before serving.

Smoked Shrimp
with Horseradish Cream

Serves 6
Carb Level: Low

Per serving:

Carbohydrate:	6.4 g
Protein:	12.6 g

This is a great do-ahead recipe.

❧

1 seedless cucumber, unpeeled
½ cup crème fraîche or sour cream
¼ cup prepared horseradish, drained and squeezed
1 tablespoon Dijon mustard
1 tablespoon fresh-squeezed lemon juice
1 teaspoon fresh chopped dill
¼ teaspoon freshly ground white pepper
Salt to taste
12–16 ounces smoked shrimp, chopped
Snipped fresh chives for garnish
Lemon wedges for garnish

1. Cut the cucumber into ½-inch slices. Use a small measuring spoon or melon baller to make a hollow in the center of each cucumber slice.
2. Mix together the crème fraîche, horseradish, Dijon, lemon juice, dill, white pepper, and salt in a bowl. Place the chopped smoked shrimp in a medium-size bowl. Add half of the horseradish dressing and toss to lightly coat. Add more dressing only if needed: be careful not to overdress.
3. Use a teaspoon to spoon a small portion of the dressed shrimp into the hollow of each cucumber slice. Top with the snipped chives. Refrigerate until ready to serve. Serve with fresh lemon wedges.

How Many Carbs in My Wine?

A bottle of wine will yield 4 to 5 servings per bottle. A bottle of champagne will yield 5 to 6 servings per bottle. A 5-ounce serving of white wine contains 1.2 grams of carbohydrates; 5 ounces of red wine contains 2.4 grams of carbohydrates; and a 5-ounce glass of champagne contains 4.3 grams of carbohydrates.

Hard-Boiled Eggs
Stuffed with Mushrooms and Cheese

1 teaspoon canola oil
½ teaspoon unsalted butter
2 shallots, minced
2 cups finely chopped button
   mushrooms
Juice of 1 lemon
1 teaspoon finely grated lemon
   zest
Salt and freshly ground black
   pepper to taste

5 large hard-boiled eggs,
   peeled
3 tablespoons mayonnaise
¼ cup shredded Gruyère
   cheese, divided
Pinch of cayenne pepper
Pinch of ground nutmeg
1 tablespoon minced fresh flat-
   leaf parsley, plus 4 extra
   leaves for garnish

Serves 4
Carb Level: Moderate

Per serving:	
Carbohydrate:	16.0 g
Protein:	14.5 g

Serve these platter style as an hors d'oeuvre or on a bed of baby greens as an appetizer.

1. Warm the oil and butter in a medium-size nonstick sauté pan over medium heat. Add the shallots and cook slowly for 3 minutes, until soft but not brown. Stir in the mushrooms, lemon juice, and lemon zest. Season with salt and black pepper. Cover and cook, stirring frequently, for 10 minutes or until the mushrooms are very soft and all the liquid has evaporated. Remove from heat.

2. Slice 4 of the hard-boiled eggs lengthwise. Remove the yolks and carefully slice a small piece from the bottom of each egg white half so that it will stand flat and steady on a platter.

3. Chop the remaining egg. Using a spatula, press it through a fine-mesh sieve into the pan with the mushrooms. Stir in the mayonnaise and add 2 tablespoons of the cheese, the cayenne, and nutmeg. Add the minced parsley, and season with salt and pepper. Cover and keep warm.

4. Preheat the oven to 375°. Place an equal portion of the mushroom mixture in each egg-white half, mounding it slightly. Place the filled egg halves in a baking dish and sprinkle the tops with the remaining Gruyère; bake for 4 minutes, then turn on the broiler (on low) and cook for about 2 minutes, until golden brown and bubbly. Serve hot.

Mussel Salad with Green Beans

Serves 4
Carb Level: Moderate

Per serving:	
Carbohydrate:	19.9 g
Protein:	23.2 g

Fresh farm-raised mussels are readily available at most fish counters.

❧

¾ pound small green beans, trimmed and cut into 1½-inch pieces
Salt
1½ pounds fresh mussels
2 teaspoons butter
3 medium shallots, minced
¼ cup dry white wine
1 large ripe tomato, peeled, seeded, cored, and diced

2 tablespoons chopped fresh flat-leaf parsley, divided
½ cup olive oil
Juice of 1 lemon
2 tablespoons rice wine vinegar
Freshly ground black pepper to taste
½ cucumber, sliced paper-thin

1. Place the green beans in a medium-size saucepan and add cold water to cover by about 1 inch. Add 1 teaspoon of salt. Bring to a boil over medium-high heat. Reduce the heat to medium-low and simmer for 3 to 5 minutes, until the beans are very tender; drain well. To stop the cooking, immediately plunge the beans in a bowl of ice water or run under very cold running water. Drain well and place in a medium-size bowl.

2. Wash the mussels very well in 3 changes of clean water. Scrub off any grit and remove the beards. Discard any open mussels.

3. Melt the butter in a large saucepan over medium heat. Add half of the shallots and sauté for 3 minutes, without browning. Add the mussels and wine, and raise the heat to high. Cover and cook for 3 minutes, or until the mussels open, shaking the pan while they are covered. Discard any mussels that do not open. Remove from heat.

4. Toss the tomato, 1 tablespoon of parsley, olive oil, lemon juice, rice wine vinegar, and remaining shallots in a small bowl; mix to combine and add salt and pepper to taste. Arrange the cucumbers around the edge of each of 4 chilled salad plates or on 1 medium-size platter. Place equal portions of the salad in the center and sprinkle with the chopped parsley. Arrange the mussels around the salad. Drizzle the vinaigrette over the beans, cucumbers, and mussels. Serve immediately. (As the green beans sit in the tossed vinegar, they will slowly begin to turn color due to the acid in the dressing. Don't dress the salad until just before serving.)

Mexican-Style Shrimp Cocktail

1 cup ketchup
²/₃ cup orange juice
2 tablespoons fresh-squeezed lime juice
2 tablespoons dry white wine
2 teaspoons Worcestershire sauce
1 teaspoon hot pepper sauce

Salt and freshly ground black pepper to taste
3 cups shrimp, cooked, peeled, and deveined
6 lime wedges for garnish

Whisk together the ketchup, orange juice, lime juice, wine, Worcestershire sauce, and hot pepper sauce in a large bowl. Season with salt and pepper. Taste and add more lime juice or salt if desired. Stir in the shrimp. Cover and marinate in the refrigerator for 5 minutes or up to 4 hours before serving. Divide the shrimp mixture among 6 martini or margarita glasses. Garnish each with a lime wedge.

Serves 6

Carb Level: Moderate

Per serving:

Carbohydrate:	14.8 g
Protein:	25.8 g

Easy to do ahead, and takes just minutes to prepare. Serve in chilled martini or margarita glasses.

❧

Orange-Cucumber Salsa

Makes 4 cups
Carb Level: Moderate

Per serving:	
Carbohydrate:	19.1 g
Protein:	2.9 g

Great as a dipping salsa or as an accompaniment to fish or shellfish.

4 large oranges
4 seedless cucumbers, washed
½ cup rice wine vinegar

2 tablespoons olive oil
1 teaspoon red pepper flakes

1. Grate the rind of 1 or 2 of the oranges to yield 1 teaspoon grated zest. Trim the rind from the oranges, including as much of the white pith as possible. Cut the oranges into segments, remove any seeds, and dice the flesh. Place the diced oranges in a medium-size bowl along with any accumulated juices. (You should have about 2 cups.)
2. Peel 2 of the cucumbers. Split all of the cucumbers lengthwise and use a small spoon to scoop out the seeds. Cut all 4 cucumbers into ¼-inch slices. (You should have about 2 cups.) Add to the bowl with the oranges.
3. Whisk together the vinegar, oil, and red pepper flakes. Pour the mixture over the top of the oranges and cucumbers and add salt and freshly ground black pepper to taste. Cover and marinate in the refrigerator for 1 to 2 hours. Serve chilled.

What Is a Tomatillo?

Tomatillo is a fruit and is also known as a Mexican green tomato. Tomatillos should be used while they are green and still quite firm. They come with a parchmentlike covering. To use tomatillos, remove the covering and wash. Tomatillos have a flavor with hints of lemon, apples, and herbs. Cooking enhances the tomatillo's flavor and softens its thick skin. Tomatillos are generally used in Mexican sauces and salsa

Stuffed Zucchini

4 large zucchini
¼ cup butter
1 shallot, chopped
2 cloves garlic, crushed
1 cup chopped button
  mushrooms
½ cup chopped spinach,
  cooked and drained
4 ounces smoked mozzarella
  cheese, grated
1 tablespoon ketchup

1 tablespoon chopped fresh
  parsley
Salt and freshly ground black
  pepper to taste
1 teaspoon honey
1 egg, beaten
½ cup toasted pine nuts

Serves 4
Carb Level: Moderate

Per serving:	
Carbohydrate:	13.6 g
Protein:	9.6 g

This recipe also works great with medium size zucchini. You can also substitute yellow summer squash.

☙

1. Trim off the ends of the zucchini, halve them lengthwise, and use a small spoon to scoop some out some of the seeded flesh to form hollow "boats." Bring a large pan of salted water to a boil and blanch the zucchini for 2 minutes. Drain well, then place them cut-side up in a greased casserole dish.

2. Heat the butter in a large saucepan over medium-high heat and sauté the shallot and garlic for 2 minutes. Add the mushrooms and spinach, and cook gently for 4 minutes to remove any liquid. Stir in the cheese, then the ketchup. Add the parsley, and season with salt and pepper; then stir in the honey. Remove the saucepan from the heat and stir in the egg and nuts.

3. Preheat oven to 400°.

4. Fill the zucchini halves with this mixture. Cook, uncovered, for about 10 minutes until heated throughout. Serve hot, with a salad of thinly sliced tomatoes as a first course, or as a buffet item.

Mushrooms Au Gratin

Serves 4

Carb Level: Moderate

Per serving:

Carbohydrate:	18.5 g
Protein:	4.5 g

An excellent side dish that can be easily made in larger quantities.

∾

*1 pound small button
  mushrooms, cleaned and
  stems trimmed
Juice of 1 lemon
2 tablespoons brandy
¼ cup vegetable oil
1 small shallot, chopped
2 tablespoons sour cream
2 tablespoons tomato paste
2 teaspoons honey*

*Salt and freshly ground black
  pepper to taste
Pinch of cayenne pepper
2 tablespoons Dijon mustard
1 tablespoon bread crumbs
2 tablespoons grated Gruyère
  cheese*

1. Put the mushrooms in a medium-size bowl and stir in the lemon juice and brandy; let marinate for 10 minutes.
2. Heat the oil in a skillet or frying pan over medium-high heat and sauté the shallot for 1 minute, without browning it. Add the marinade juices to the shallot and cook for 2 minutes to reduce the liquid.
3. Add the mushrooms and cook for 2 minutes. Remove them from the skillet with a slotted spoon and keep warm in a shallow ovenproof dish. Add the sour cream, tomato paste, honey, salt and pepper, and cayenne to the skillet juices, stir to mix, and boil for 2 minutes to reduce further. Stir in the mustard but do not allow the sauce to boil.
4. Preheat the broiler on low.
5. Pour the sauce over the mushrooms. Combine the bread crumbs and cheese, and sprinkle over the mushrooms. Brown under a broiler until golden. Serve on a platter with toothpicks on the side.

Stewed Pepper and Tomato Purée

4 red bell peppers
2 tablespoons olive oil
2 cloves garlic, quartered
1 teaspoon salt
Red chili pepper flakes to taste

1 cup tomato sauce
1 tablespoon tomato paste

Serves 4
Carb Level: Moderate

Per serving:	
Carbohydrate:	19.3 g
Protein:	3.1 g

Spoon 1 or 2 table-spoons on the center of a dinner plate before serving with a simple grilled or roasted meat or fish.

1. Quarter the peppers; cut off the stems, and remove the seeds and the inner membrane. Chop the peppers into large pieces.
2. Heat the oil on medium-high in a nonstick sauté pan; stew the peppers with the garlic over low heat until very soft. Season with salt and red chili flakes.
3. Transfer the peppers and garlic to a food processor or blender; process until puréed. Return the pepper mixture to the sauté pan and add the tomato sauce and tomato paste; stir to mix, and bring to a light simmer. Serve hot.

A Variation for Chicken

Whisk in a couple of tablespoons of goat cheese to the hot sauce to make a great sauce for chicken.

Eggplant Topped with Gruyère Cheese

Serves 4
Carb Level: Moderate
Per serving:
Carbohydrate: 14.4 g
Protein: 19.3 g

A tasty dish to satisfy cravings for a deep-fried dish.

∾

2 large eggplants
Salt
5 cups vegetable oil
1 clove garlic, minced
8 ounces Gruyère cheese or
  mozzarella cheese, thinly
  sliced

Chopped fresh parsley for
  garnish

1. Cut the eggplants crosswise into slices ½-inch thick. Sprinkle each slice with salt and let sit for 25 minutes (this extracts the bitter-tasting juices). Rinse under cold running water, drain, and dry thoroughly.
2. Preheat broiler on low.
3. Heat the oil and deep-fry each eggplant slice for 1 minute. Drain on paper towels. Arrange the slices in a single layer on a flat baking sheet, sprinkle with the garlic, and place a slice of cheese over each slice. Broil until the cheese is bubbly and golden. Sprinkle with a little chopped parsley and serve immediately.

Avocado and Tomato Dip

2 ripe avocados
2 tomatoes, peeled, seeded,
    and chopped
1 tablespoon tomato paste
Juice and grated rind of
    1 lemon
1 clove garlic
1 small onion, chopped
2 tablespoons chopped fresh
    parsley

8 ounces cottage cheese
1 teaspoon salt
Pinch of paprika
Freshly ground black pepper

Serves 4
Carb Level: Moderate

Per serving:	
Carbohydrate:	18.7 g
Protein:	10.6 g

Use this as a dip for vegetables or as a topping for shellfish—also pairs well with shrimp and lobster dishes.

1. To peel the avocado, make a slice lengthwise around the center of the pit; twist the halves apart. To remove the pit, poke a fork into the seed and twist. Smash the avocado flesh with the back of a fork until somewhat creamy.
2. In a blender or food processor, blend together the tomatoes, tomato paste, lemon juice, lemon rind, garlic, onion, parsley and cottage cheese. In a large bowl, combine all the ingredients together and stir, seasoning with salt, paprika, and pepper. Serve chilled or at room temperature. Note that avocados will turn brown as they sit out. This dish should be prepared just before serving.

Spicy Olive and Walnut Tapenade

2 cups large black pitted kalamata olives, drained
1 ¾ cups shelled walnuts
¼ cup large capers
2 tablespoons sour cream
1 teaspoon red chili pepper
  flakes
4 hard-boiled eggs, peeled and
  quartered

2 cloves garlic
2 tablespoons soy sauce
1 tablespoon chopped parsley
2 tablespoons red wine vinegar
¼ cup olive oil
Pinch of dried tarragon
1 teaspoon honey
Salt and freshly ground black
  pepper to taste

Place all the ingredients in a blender or food processor and blend to a paste. Adjust seasoning to taste. Use as a filling for vegetables or as an hors d'oeuvre. Add a small amount of cream to thin if using as a dip for vegetables.

Crab Salad

½ pound cooked, cold crabmeat, picked over for shells
3–4 tablespoons mayonnaise
Juice of 1 lemon

1 shallot, minced
Salt and freshly ground black
  pepper to taste

Combine all the ingredients in a medium-size bowl, mixing well. Adjust seasoning to taste. Serve as a centerpiece in a bed of crispy spring greens with a light citrus vinaigrette.

Canned Versus Fresh

You can use canned crabmeat for ease and convenience, but the taste difference using fresh jumbo lump crabmeat is exceptional. Be prepared for the price of fresh meat—it is expensive.

Green Beans
with Shallots and Rosemary

*1 pound green beans, ends
 trimmed*
2 tablespoons butter
*1/3 cup shallots, chopped
 (about 3 large)*

*1 teaspoon chopped fresh
 rosemary*
*Salt and freshly ground black
 pepper to taste*

Serves 5	
Carb Level: Low	
Per serving:	
Carbohydrate:	8.3 g
Protein:	2.0 g

Use fresh green
beans, which are
available in abun-
dance all year long.

❧

1. Cook the green beans in a large pot of boiling salted water until crisp-tender, about 5 minutes. Drain and rinse with cold running water until the green beans are no longer warm; drain again. Pat dry with paper towels.
2. Melt the butter in a large heavy skillet over medium-high heat. Add the shallots and rosemary, and sauté until the shallots are tender, about 5 minutes. Add the green beans and toss until heated through, about 5 minutes. Season with salt and pepper. Transfer the green beans to a bowl and serve immediately.

No Chafing Dish? No Problem.

It is not necessary to have a formal chafing dish to serve hot foods. Variations are available, but be very careful for fire hazards. Consider using a tea light setup from a fondue pot to keep soups and sauces hot. Six bricks and one sterno can also be set up as a build-your-own chafer. Always make sure there is an ovenproof plate or trivet under the sterno to prevent scorching furniture. Always check and double check the pans to make sure that they are balanced and will not tip if bumped during service.

Chicken Pâté

Serves 10
Carb Level: Low

Per serving:

Carbohydrate:	3.0 g
Protein:	11.4 g

This classic French recipe gets easier each time you make it.

∾

1 pound boneless, skinless
   chicken breasts
2 large egg whites
1/3 cup sour cream
2 tablespoons brandy

Salt and freshly ground white
   pepper
4 sprigs fresh tarragon
1/3 cup pistachio nuts, crushed
10 cups water

1. Cut the chicken into small pieces. Place 3/4 of the chicken in a food processor. Add the egg whites, sour cream, and brandy. Season with salt and pepper. Process until the mixture is very smooth. Transfer to a medium-size bowl. Strip the leaves from the tarragon and add to the bowl; discard the tarragon stems. Fold in the pistachios and the reserved chicken pieces. Place a small sauté pan on medium heat and cook about a tablespoon of the chicken mixture thoroughly. Cool slightly and taste paying particular attention to seasoning. Add more salt and pepper as needed.

2. Bring the water to a boil over high heat. Reduce the heat to medium-low. Place a large sheet of parchment (not wax paper) on a flat surface. Mound the chicken mixture on the paper in a neat log shape approximately 2" × 10", positioning it about 3 inches from the long edge of the paper. Fold the 3 inches of paper over the chicken mixture. Roll the paper around the chicken to form a neat cylinder. Twist the ends closed and tie firmly with butcher's twine.

3. Place the cylinder on a large piece of plastic wrap. Use the same technique to enclose the cylinder. Tie the ends with butcher's twine. Place in the saucepan of simmering water. Place a Pyrex dish over the cylinder to keep it submerged. Simmer for 20 minutes. Carefully, with a pair of tongs, remove the cylinder and allow to cool on a wire rack at room temperature.

4. Unwrap the log. Cut crosswise into 1/4-inch slices. Arrange the slices in a decorative pattern on a chilled serving plate with whole grain and Dijon mustards on the side, or our Spicy Olive and Walnut Tapenade (see recipe on page 268) on the side.

Tuna Tapenade

1 (3½-ounce) can albacore tuna
    packed in water, well drained
¼ cup cream cheese, at room
    temperature
2 tablespoons mayonnaise
1 tablespoon sour cream
1 tablespoon fresh-squeezed
    lemon juice

Freshly ground white pepper
1 cup fresh baby spinach leaves
½ cup chopped scallions
2 tablespoons capers, well
    drained
1 tablespoon chopped fresh dill

In a food processor, combine the tuna, cream cheese, mayonnaise, sour cream, lemon juice, and pepper; process until well blended. Add the spinach, scallions, capers, and dill; pulse again until well blended. Serve as a spread for vegetables or as a garnish on a salad of mixed greens and a simple vinaigrette.

Serves 10	
Carb Level: Low	
Per serving:	
Carbohydrate:	1.5 g
Protein:	4.5 g

A versatile spread or salad garnish that requires no cooking.

∾

Shrimp Scampi

¾ cup extra-virgin olive oil
2 large cloves garlic, slivered
1 pound large shrimp, tail on,
    shelled and deveined
2 large cloves garlic, minced
2 dried hot chili peppers

1 tablespoon grated orange zest
¼ cup minced fresh parsley
Salt and freshly ground black
    pepper to taste
1 tablespoon dry sherry

Warm the olive oil in a large skillet over medium-low heat. Add the slivered garlic and cook gently until soft and just starting to color, stirring occasionally. Place the shrimp in the pan in a single layer. Add the minced garlic, chili pepper, and orange zest. Cook, undisturbed, for 1 to 2 minutes. When the shrimp are pink on 1 side, turn them over. Add the parsley, salt and pepper, and sherry, raise the heat slightly, and cook until all the shrimp are pink, about 2 minutes more. Serve immediately.

Serves 4	
Carb Level: Low	
Per serving:	
Carbohydrate:	2.3 g
Protein:	23.4 g

Chili peppers and orange zest give this version of shrimp scampi a kick.

∾

Salmon Fillets with Basil

Serves 4
Carb Level: Low

Per serving:

Carbohydrate:	5.7 g
Protein:	36.3 g

Use only fresh salmon and buy your basil at the Farmer's Market during the summer when it's the cheapest, yet most flavorful.

∾

2 lemons
4 (6-ounce) salmon fillets, cleaned and boned
4 tablespoons unsalted butter, cut into 6 pieces
2 tablespoons olive oil
1 tablespoon shallots
2 teaspoons minced garlic
1 cup stemmed and torn fresh basil leaves
Pinch of cayenne pepper

Salt and freshly ground black pepper to taste
1 cup heavy cream, room temperature
1/4 cup coarsely chopped fresh basil for garnish

1. Squeeze 1 lemon over the salmon, making sure to coat both sides. Melt 2 tablespoons of butter and the oil over medium heat in a sauté pan large enough to accommodate the 4 fillets. When the butter and oil starts to foam, add the fillets. Cook for 3 to 5 minutes on each side; transfer to an ovenproof plate in a 200° oven.

2. Add the remaining butter to the pan, a piece at a time, and melt until foaming. Add the shallots and garlic, and cook until soft, about 2 minutes. Add the juice from the other lemon, the basil leaves, cayenne, and salt and pepper; stir to combine well. Add the heavy cream very slowly to prevent curdling, and bring to a simmer. Cook until the sauce is reduced by a third. Adjust the seasonings to taste.

3. Place the fish on warm plates or a platter with a small pool of sauce underneath each fillet. Top each lightly with a little more sauce and sprinkle with the basil.

Scallops in an Herbed Tomato Sauce

¼ cup butter
1 clove garlic, minced
1 shallot, minced
1½ cups chopped tomatoes
*   (canned or fresh)*
1 teaspoon balsamic vinegar
2 tablespoons red wine
Salt and freshly ground black
*   pepper to taste*
1 teaspoon fresh tarragon,
*   minced, or 1 teaspoon dried*

1 teaspoon fresh thyme leaves
1 pound large sea scallops,
*   hinges on the side of each*
*   scallop removed*
1–2 tablespoons olive oil
Fresh basil, minced, for garnish

Serves 4
Carb Level: Low

Per serving:	
Carbohydrate:	7.3 g
Protein:	19.9 g

You can substitute fish such as cod, grouper, or snapper for the scallops in this recipe.

ɑ

1. Melt half of the butter in a small saucepan over medium heat until foamy; cook the garlic and shallot, stirring occasionally, until softened. Add the tomatoes and cook about 10 minutes, stirring occasionally. Stir in the vinegar, wine, salt and pepper, tarragon, thyme, and the remaining butter. Cool slightly and purée in a blender or food processor; keep warm.

2. Heat a 12-inch nonstick skillet over high heat until almost smoking. Place the scallops on a plate, sprinkle them with some salt, and brush or drizzle them with a little olive oil. Add the scallops to the pan 1 at a time; turn them as they brown, allowing about 2 minutes on each side. Pour a little sauce onto each of four plates or a large platter and top with the scallops and basil.

Beef with Cucumber

Serves 4

Carb Level: Low

Per serving:

Carbohydrate:	4.9 g
Protein:	27.2 g

For presentation as an appetizer, serve the steak on mini-skewers.

8 ounces plain yogurt
¼ cup cucumber, coarsely shredded and unpeeled
1 tablespoon finely chopped red onion
1 tablespoon coarsely chopped fresh mint
¼ teaspoon sugar

Salt and freshly ground black pepper to taste
1 pound (1-inch-thick) boneless beef sirloin steak
½ teaspoon lemon-pepper seasoning
Mint leaves for garnish

1. Preheat a gas grill or broiler. Make sure the grill grate is clean and lightly oiled to prevent sticking.
2. Combine the yogurt, cucumber, onion, mint, and sugar in a small bowl. Season to taste with salt and pepper; set aside.
3. Trim the fat from the steak. Sprinkle the steak with salt and lemon-pepper seasoning on both sides. Grill the steak on the rack of an uncovered grill directly over medium heat or broil for 12 to 15 minutes for medium, turning once. Let the steak sit at room temperature for 5 minutes before carving. Using a long straight-edge slicing knife, cut the steak into thin strips across the grain of the meat. Roll each slice and secure with a toothpick and place on a platter that is garnished with mint leaves. Serve the cucumber raita sauce on the side.

Eat Often

Don't ever go longer than 6 hours without having a protein meal or protein-rich snack. "Fasting" will cause you to crave sugars. Planning your meal and snacks will allow you to better manage your diet plan.

Chicken with Nectarine Salsa

4 large boneless, skinless
   chicken breasts halves
   (about 1 pound total)
1 tablespoon lime juice
1–1½ teaspoons ground cumin
Salt and freshly ground black
   pepper to taste
½ cup chunky salsa
⅓ cup chopped nectarine

2 tablespoons chopped fresh
   cilantro
1 jalapeño, seeded and finely
   chopped
1 teaspoon minced garlic
Lime wedges for garnish

Serves 4
Carb Level: Low

Per serving:	
Carbohydrate:	5.0 g
Protein:	32.6 g

Adding a small amount of fresh, ripe fruit to a quality premade salsa is a great time-saver. Also try peaches, mangos, or citrus fruits.

1. Preheat a gas grill or broiler. Make sure the grill grate is clean and lightly oiled to prevent sticking.
2. Rinse the chicken and pat dry. Brush the chicken with lime juice and sprinkle evenly with cumin and salt and pepper. Grill the chicken on the rack of an uncovered grill directly over medium heat or broil for 12 to 15 minutes, until the chicken is tender and no longer pink, turning once.
3. For the nectarine salsa, stir together the salsa, nectarine, cilantro, jalapeño, and garlic in a small bowl; spoon over the chicken, and serve with the lime wedges on the side for garnish.

Cooking Chicken Safely

Chicken must be cooked to the following internal temperatures to insure food safety and proper elimination of bacteria.

Boneless chicken	165°
Bone-in chicken pieces	170°
Ground chicken	165°
Bone-in whole chicken	180°

Sautéed Spinach with Pine Nuts

Serves 2
Carb Level: Low

Per serving:	
Carbohydrate:	6.4 g
Protein:	1.6 g

The sesame oil and bouillon granules add a twist to traditional sautéed spinach.

❧

1 tablespoon pine nuts
1 tablespoon olive oil
¼ cup chopped yellow onion
1 clove garlic, chopped
2 tablespoons rice wine
⅛ teaspoon dark sesame oil
½ teaspoon chicken bouillon
   granules

Freshly ground black pepper to
   taste
5 ounces (about 1 bunch)
   fresh spinach, washed,
   stemmed, and chopped
1 teaspoon lemon juice

1. Toast the pine nuts in a small skillet over low heat, turning often, until lightly browned (2 minutes or so); set aside.
2. Heat the oil in a large skillet over medium heat; add the onion and cook until soft, about 4 minutes. Add the garlic and cook for another minute. Stir in the rice wine, sesame oil, bouillon granules, and pepper. Add the spinach and reduce the heat to medium-low. Cover and cook until tender, about 6 minutes. Stir in the lemon juice; cook for 1 minute. Stir in the pine nuts and adjust seasoning to taste. Serve immediately on a serving platter or in a bowl.

Roasting Veggies the Right Way

Roasted vegetable platters are a great "do-ahead" dish and a colorful way to serve an assortment of delicious tasting vegetables. The key is to start with a very hot oven—400° to 450° degrees is ideal. Toss the vegetables with a small amount of olive oil and season liberally with pepper and Kosher salt and place on a baking sheet in a single layer. Place in the oven and turn the vegetables frequently, about every 3 minutes until just starting to caramelize on the outside but not overcooked. The vegetables should still have shape and texture. Roast each type of vegetable individually; mising them all together to cook muddies the flavors. Roasted vegetables can be served warm or at room temperature.

Grilled Tomatoes

6 large ripe tomatoes
2 teaspoons olive oil
Salt and freshly ground black
*   pepper to taste*

1 tablespoon fresh thyme

Preheat a grill or grill pan to high (grill pan should be almost smoking). Make sure the grill grates are clean and lightly oiled to prevent sticking. Halve the tomatoes crosswise. Gently squeeze each half to remove the seeds. Lightly brush the tomatoes with the oil and season with salt and pepper. Place, cut-side down, on the hottest part of the grill; grill for 1 minute. Turn the tomatoes, moving them to the edge of the grill or to wherever the heat is reduced. Grill for 3 minutes or until charred. Remove from the grill and season with the fresh thyme. Serve warm or at room temperature.

Serves 12
Carb Level: Low

Per serving:

Carbohydrate:	2.9 g
Protein:	0.5 g

Sprinkle a little grated Parmesan cheese over the tops as soon as they come off the grill to enhance the tomato and fresh herb flavors.

Grilled Radicchio

3 heads radicchio
1 tablespoon extra-virgin
*   olive oil*
Salt and freshly ground black
*   pepper to taste*

Freshly grated Parmesan cheese
*   (optional)*

Preheat a gas grill or a griddle pan to low. Make sure the grill grate is clean and lightly oiled to prevent sticking. Remove any damaged outer leaves from the radicchio. Trim the stem and quarter the radicchio lengthwise, leaving the core intact. Lightly brush with the oil and season with salt and pepper. Place on the grill; grill for 8 minutes or until tender and lightly browned. Serve warm or at room temperature. If you like, drizzle a touch more olive oil over it and sprinkle with grated Parmesan cheese.

Serves 12
Carb Level: Low

Per serving:

Carbohydrate:	0.1 g
Protein:	0.0 g

For a richer, sweeter taste, blanch the radicchio in lightly salted water for 1 minute, then drain well and grill.

CHAPTER 16

Holiday Dishes

Thanksgiving

Oven-Roasted Winter Vegetables ❖	280
Pear and Pumpkin Soup ❖	281
Sautéed Green Beans with Shiitake Mushrooms ❖	282
Cornbread Stuffing ❖	283
Rosemary Jus	284

Hanukkah

Smoked Whitefish Salad ❖	285
Braised Brisket ❖	286
Matzo Ball Soup	287
Chopped Liver ❖	288

New Year's Eve

Celery Root and Pear Purée ❖	289
Beet Dip ❖	290
Turkey Meatballs with Tomato Sauce ❖	291
Beef Tenderloin in a Red Wine–Peppercorn Sauce	292
Oysters Rockefeller Soup	293
Lobster in Vanilla Sauce	294

Christmas

Glazed Carrots with Balsamic Vinegar ❖	295
Glazed Baked Ham with Rosemary	295
Butternut Squash and Turnip Gratin with Gruyère	296
Fennel- and Garlic-Crusted Pork Roast	297

Fourth of July

Spicy Chilled Shrimp ❖	298
Egg Salad with Endive Leaves ❖	298
Chili Cheese Corn Casserole ❖	299
Spicy Cucumber Relish ❖	299
Tandoori Chicken Kebabs ❖	300
Grilled Beef and Onion Kebabs ❖	301

❖ **Indicates Easy Recipe** ❖

Oven-Roasted Winter Vegetables

Serves 6

Carb Level: Moderate

Per serving:

Carbohydrate:	20.0 g
Protein:	3.1 g

This colorful dish can be easily increased for larger parties.

∾

½ pound rutabagas, peeled and cut into 1-inch pieces

½ pound carrots, peeled and cut into 1-inch pieces

½ pound parsnips, peeled and cut into 1-inch pieces

½ pound Brussels sprouts, trimmed

1 tablespoon unsalted butter

1 tablespoon extra-virgin olive oil

2 teaspoons chopped fresh thyme

2 teaspoons chopped fresh sage

⅛ teaspoon freshly grated nutmeg

Salt and freshly ground black pepper to taste

½ cup Marsala wine

1. Preheat oven to 450°.
2. Bring a large pot of salted water to a boil. Add the rutabagas, carrots, and parsnips, and simmer until they are somewhat tender when pierced with a fork, about 5 to 8 minutes. Drain well.
3. Place the rutabagas, carrots, parsnips, and Brussels sprouts in a large roasting pan. Melt the butter in a small saucepan and stir in the oil, thyme, sage, and nutmeg. Drizzle the butter mixture over the vegetables and toss to coat them completely. Season with salt and pepper. Pour the Marsala into the bottom of the roasting pan.
4. Cover tightly with foil and bake in the oven for 40 minutes. Remove the foil, toss the vegetables, and continue to cook, uncovered, until the Marsala is evaporated and the vegetables can easily be pierced with a knife, 20 to 30 minutes. Place the roasted vegetables on a platter and serve immediately.

Pear and Pumpkin Soup

½ cup chopped onion
½ cup chicken stock
1 (16-ounce) can pumpkin
    purée
2½ cups half-and-half
1¾ cups pear nectar
¼ teaspoon ground ginger

¼ teaspoon freshly ground
    white pepper
Salt to taste

1. Combine the onion and chicken stock in a large saucepan; bring to a boil. Reduce heat and simmer, covered, for about 10 minutes or until the onion is very tender; let cool slightly.
2. Transfer the mixture to a blender or food processor. Add the pumpkin, cover, and blend until smooth. Return the pumpkin mixture to the saucepan. Stir in the half-and-half, pear nectar, ginger, and white pepper. Cook and stir until heated through. Taste and season with salt if needed. Ladle into soup bowls.

Serves 6
Carb Level: Moderate
Per serving:

Carbohydrate:	20.0 g
Protein:	4.2 g

Top this dish with 2 very thin pear slices or a dollop of sour cream just before you serve.

~

The Two Types of Dietary Fiber

Insoluble fiber is found in whole grains and other plants. It absorbs water and creates peristalsis, the natural contraction of your intestinal wall to move solid materials through the digestive tract. Soluble fiber is found in forms such as pectin (in apples) and beta-glucans (in oats and barley). A diet high in soluble fiber helps reduce cholesterol, which offers protection against heart disease.

Sautéed Green Beans with Shiitake Mushrooms

Serves 8
Carb Level: Moderate

Per serving:	
Carbohydrate:	12.7 g
Protein:	3.5 g

You can substitute domestic button mushrooms to lower the carb count, but don't expect the same complex flavor and textures.

ɤ

2 pounds green beans, stemmed

3 tablespoons olive oil

1 pound Shitake mushrooms, thinly sliced

1 small red onion, thinly sliced

2 cloves garlic, minced

¼ cup rice wine

1 teaspoon chopped fresh thyme leaves

2 tablespoons unsalted butter, softened

Salt and freshly ground black pepper to taste

1. Prepare a large bowl of ice water; set aside. Bring a large pot of salted water to a rolling boil. Add the green beans and cook for 4 to 5 minutes, until crisp-tender. Drain the green beans, then submerge them in the ice water for 2 to 3 minutes. Drain well.

2. In a large nonstick skillet, heat the olive oil over medium-high heat. Add the mushrooms, onion, and garlic; cook, stirring occasionally, until the mushrooms are nicely browned, about 10 to 11 minutes. Add the rice wine, and cook for 1 minute.

3. Add the green beans and thyme, and cook until heated through. Remove from the heat, add the butter, and toss to combine. Season to taste with salt and pepper. Serve warm.

Managing Carbs During the Holidays

Focus on foods that you can have, not those that you can't. It is more powerful to think "substitute" instead of "eliminate."

Cornbread Stuffing

1 cup white or yellow
   cornmeal
1 cup all-purpose flour
2 tablespoons sugar
1 tablespoon baking powder
1/4 teaspoon baking soda
1/4 teaspoon salt
1 1/4 cups buttermilk or whole
   milk

1/4 cup unsalted butter, melted
1/4 cup vegetable oil
1 large egg

Serves 8
Carb Level: Moderate

Per serving:	
Carbohydrate:	17.8 g
Protein:	12.1 g

Tastes best when eaten the same day it's made—allow it to cool, covered, in the refrigerator until ready to serve.

❧

1. Preheat the oven to 350°. Butter an 8-inch square baking pan.
2. In a large bowl, whisk together the cornmeal, flour, sugar, baking powder, baking soda, and salt.
3. In another bowl, whisk together the buttermilk, melted butter, oil, and egg until smooth. Stir the wet into the dry ingredients, and when smooth and well mixed, pour the batter into the prepared pan. Bake for 35 to 40 minutes, or until a toothpick inserted near the center comes out clean and the cornbread begins to pull away from the sides of the pan, and the top is golden brown. Cool in the pan set on a wire rack. When cool, crumble into large pieces. Stuff into your turkey that has been baked halfway or serve just as is.

Rosemary Jus

Serves 8
Carb Level: Low

Per serving:	
Carbohydrate:	9.9 g
Protein:	2.2 g

A delicious accompaniment to the sliced turkey.

Turkey wing tips, neck, and giblets, reserved from the turkey (about 2 cups total)
8 cups turkey or chicken stock
3 sprigs fresh rosemary
1 tablespoon cornstarch stirred into 2 tablespoons cold water

Salt and freshly ground white pepper to taste
1/4 cup butter, cut into pieces

1. Chop the turkey neck into large pieces. Transfer the neck pieces to a large, heavy saucepan and add the giblets, wing tips, and stock. Bring to a boil over medium-high heat, skimming any impurities that foam and accumulate at the top. Reduce the heat to low and simmer for 3 hours.

2. Strain the stock through a strainer into a bowl. Chop the meat from the neck and the giblets and transfer to a small bowl. Cover and refrigerate. Discard the bones. Pour the pan drippings from the turkey into a bowl. Skim off and discard the fat that rises to the surface and set the drippings aside.

3. Set the roasting pan over 2 burners and add 2 cups of the strained turkey stock (not the drippings). Bring to a boil and use a wooden spoon to scrape up any browned bits sticking to the bottom of the pan. Transfer the stock to a saucepan and add the reserved pan drippings, remaining stock, and rosemary. Bring to a boil over high heat and cook until reduced to about 4 cups and the sauce is richly flavored. Whisk in the cornstarch mixture, if necessary, to thicken. Cook for about 2 minutes. Add the reserved meat and giblets, and season with salt and pepper. Whisk in the butter to enrich the sauce. Serve hot from the stove.

Smoked Whitefish Salad

¼ medium yellow onion, finely
  chopped
½ whole smoked whitefish
  (about 2 pounds)
1 hard-boiled egg, finely
  chopped
¾ cup mayonnaise

1 tablespoon fresh-squeezed
  lemon juice
1 tablespoon Dijon mustard
Salt and freshly ground black
  pepper to taste

Serves 4	
Carb Level: Low	
Per serving:	
Carbohydrate:	4.2 g
Protein:	2.5 g

Smoked whitefish is usually available at your local Jewish deli.

∽

1. Place the chopped onion in a small bowl and cover with ice water. Let soak for 15 minutes. Drain and pat dry.
2. Use a small knife and your fingertips to remove and discard the skin, bones, and any brown bits from the whitefish. Gently sort through the meat to ensure all small bones have been removed. Flake the whitefish into small pieces into a medium-size bowl, checking again for any bones.
3. Add the egg and onion to the whitefish and mash together with a fork. Blend in the mayonnaise, lemon juice, and Dijon. (For a smoother salad, pulse the whitefish mixture in a food processor.) Season with salt and pepper to taste. Serve immediately or store in the refrigerator for up to 3 days.

Avoiding Caffeine

Avoid coffee, tea, and soft drinks with caffeine. Caffeine can lower your blood sugar, causing you to crave sugar and sweets. This is key during the holidays where there is an overabundance of candy and dessert items.

Braised Brisket

Serves 8
Carb Level: Moderate

Per serving:	
Carbohydrate:	16.3 g
Protein:	50.4 g

This recipe is best when it's allowed to sit overnight in its own juices.

∾

5 pounds beef brisket, first
    cut, trimmed
3 tablespoons canola oil
Salt and freshly ground black
    pepper to taste
3 pounds onions, thinly sliced
6 medium carrots, peeled and
    cut into a large dice
5 cloves garlic, crushed

2 teaspoons peppercorns
Beef stock to cover brisket,
    approximately 3–4 cups
Fresh parsley, chopped,
    for garnish

1. Preheat oven to 325°.
2. Pat the brisket with paper towels to dry. Heat the oil in a Dutch oven on high heat. Season the meat with salt and pepper. Brown the meat on all sides, then remove from the Dutch oven. Add the onions and carrots to the Dutch oven, and sauté until golden. Return the meat to the pan and add the garlic and peppercorns. Add beef stock just to cover the brisket. Bring just to a boil, cover, and place in the oven for at least 3 hours.
3. Season with salt and pepper, slice, and serve with its own juice. Garnish with the parsley.

Slicing Braised Brisket

Braised brisket is very tender. To make it easier to cut into slices without it falling apart, use a very sharp slicing knife after the beef is chilled thoroughly from the refrigerator. Once the chilled beef is sliced, gently reheat with a small amount of the braising juices.

Matzo Ball Soup

Soup:

1 whole roasting chicken
3 whole carrots, cut into large
    chunks
4 celery sticks (stalks and
    tops), cut into large chunks
2 whole onions, quartered
½ cup chopped fresh parsley
1 parsnip, peeled and cut into
    large chunks
4 sprigs fresh dill
Salt and freshly ground black
    pepper to taste

Matzo Balls:

3 large eggs, separated
2 tablespoons chicken fat or
    vegetable oil
½ cup matzo meal
1 teaspoon salt
2 tablespoons soup stock
    (from above) or water

Serves 12

Carb Level: Low

Per serving:	
Carbohydrate:	7.6 g
Protein:	23.5 g

This traditional soup tastes best when made the day before serving. Gently reheat the matzo balls in a small amount of the soup before serving.

~

---

1. To prepare the soup: Use kitchen shears to cut the whole chicken into quarters. Place the chicken into a stockpot and fill the stockpot with water to cover chicken. Bring the stockpot to a boil. Skim off any impurities that rise to the top of the water. Add the rest of the ingredients for the soup. Reduce heat and let simmer, partially covered, for approximately 1½ hours or until tender.

2. To prepare the matzo balls: Mix the egg yolks with the chicken fat (or oil) in a medium-size mixing bowl. Mix together the matzo meal, salt, and soup stock; add to the egg yolk mixture, and stir to blend. Beat the egg whites to soft peaks. Fold the egg whites into the matzo mixture until just blended, and refrigerate for 40 minutes. Remove from the refrigerator and make heaping tablespoon-size balls.

3. Strain the soup, reserving the chicken for another use. Reserve the carrots. Put the strained soup back into the stockpot, bring back to a low boil, and carefully drop the matzo balls into the soup. Cover and simmer for about 40 minutes. Serve the matzo ball soup in warmed soup cups with a few slices of the reserved carrots.

Chopped Liver

Serves 4
Carb Level: Low

Per serving:	
Carbohydrate:	5.4 g
Protein:	13.8 g

Every family has their own version, but the ingredients for traditional chopped liver are pretty much standard.

∾

1 large onion, chopped
3 tablespoons chicken fat or vegetable oil
1–2 eggs
½ pound chicken livers

Salt and freshly ground black pepper to taste

1. Fry the onion in the chicken fat (*or* oil) on low heat in a large frying pan with the lid on, until very soft and golden, stirring occasionally. Let cool.
2. Hard-boil the eggs by bringing them to a boil for 9 minutes, then cool them under running water.
3. Preheat the broiler. Line a baking sheet with aluminum foil.
4. Rinse the livers, pat dry, and sprinkle with salt. Put the livers on the baking sheet in a single layer and cook briefly, turning once, until they change color and are cooked through. Let them cool.
5. Cut the hard-boiled eggs in half and chop them finely in a food processor; transfer them to a mixing bowl. Reserve 2 to 3 tablespoons of chopped egg to use as a garnish. Transfer the livers and onions to the workbowl of a food processor. Pulse briefly, leaving the paste a little coarse. Mix the liver and onions with the rest of the chopped eggs by hand. Season with salt and pepper and mix well. Smooth the surface flat and sprinkle with the chopped egg.

Celery Root and Pear Purée

*1 large celery root, peeled and
   cut into 1-inch cubes*
½ large white onion, diced
*2 ripe Anjou pears, peeled,
   cored, and diced*
¾ cup heavy cream
3 tablespoons unsalted butter

*Salt and freshly ground black
   pepper to taste*
*Fresh watercress leaves for
   garnish*
*Crumbled goat cheese for
   garnish*

Serves 4
Carb Level: Moderate

Per serving:

Carbohydrate:	19.1 g
Protein:	2.2 g

Makes a wonderful
starter course to a
holiday meal.

1. Place the celery root, onion, and pears in a medium-size saucepan and covered with water; bring to a boil over high heat. Reduce the heat to a simmer and cook until the celery root is very soft, about 50 minutes. Drain, reserving ½ cup of the cooking liquid.
2. Place the celery root mixture in a blender or food processor and process until smooth. Add the cream, butter, salt, and pepper; pulse to combine. If necessary, reheat over low heat, stirring frequently. If the mixture seems too thick, add a little of the reserved cooking liquid. Adjust seasoning to taste. Garnish with watercress leaves and goat cheese. Serve hot.

Love Garlic?

Garlic is a wonderful flavoring agent. You can estimate about 1 gram of carbohydrate for 1 average size clove of garlic. When using chopped garlic in a sautéed dish, be careful not to burn or allow the garlic to get too brown as it will impart a bitter taste to your dish.

Beet Dip

Serves 10
Carb Level: Low

Per serving:

Carbohydrate:	8.1 g
Protein:	2.3 g

Serve with spears of Belgian endive layed out from the center of the platter for a festive presentation.

☙

6 fresh red beets
Splash of vinegar, lemon juice,
   or red wine
1 cup chopped red onion
¾ cup sour cream
¾ cup plain yogurt
¾ cup chopped fresh dill

4 large cloves garlic, minced
Salt and freshly ground black
   pepper to taste

1. Cook the beets in large pot of boiling salted water, with a splash of vinegar, lemon juice, *or* red wine added, until tender, about 35 minutes. Drain, and let cool. Peel and chop coarsely. (You may want to wear rubber gloves while peeling, as the beets will stain your fingers.)
2. Combine the beets and onion in a blender or food processor; blend until smooth. Transfer the beet mixture to a medium-size bowl and mix in the sour cream, yogurt, dill, and garlic. Season the dip to taste with salt and pepper. Cover and refrigerate for up to 2 days. Spoon the dip into a bowl and serve chilled.

Creating a Cheese Board

Cheese boards are an easy and elegant entertaining style. A cheese board should include a mix of goat, cow, and sheep's milk cheese. Use a variety of textures including soft cheeses such as Brie or camembert; smoked cheeses such as mozzarella, gouda, or provolone; hard cheeses such as manchego; and blue cheeses such as Roquefort or gorgonzola.

Turkey Meatballs with Tomato Sauce

2 tablespoons butter
1 slightly beaten egg white
¼ cup fine dry bread crumbs
2 tablespoons plain nonfat
   yogurt
2 tablespoons chopped fresh
   basil
¼ teaspoon freshly ground
   black pepper

12 ounces ground raw turkey
1 (16-ounce) can tomatoes,
   undrained
3 tablespoons tomato paste
½ teaspoon sugar
⅛ teaspoon salt

Makes 36 Meatballs	
Carb Level: Low	
Per serving:	
Carbohydrate:	3.0 g
Protein:	4.3 g

A great dish to serve at parties.

1. Preheat oven to 400°. Spray a shallow baking pan with nonstick coating.
2. Combine the butter, egg white, bread crumbs, yogurt, half the basil, and the pepper in a medium-size bowl. Add the ground turkey, and mix well. Shape into 1-inch meatballs (should yield 36 meatballs). Place in the prepared pan and bake for about 20 minutes or until no pink remains.
3. Meanwhile, for the sauce, combine the tomatoes and their liquid, the tomato paste, the remaining basil, sugar, and salt in a blender or food processor. Cover, and blend just until mixed and tomatoes are slightly chunky. Transfer the mixture to a medium-size saucepan; bring to a boil. Reduce heat and simmer, uncovered, for 10 to 15 minutes or to desired consistency. Serve the meatballs on wooden picks with tomato sauce for dipping.

Entertaining with Olives

Olives are a favorite during the holiday entertaining season. Instead of serving tapanades, which require a chip, consider serving quality imported olives that have been marinated with peppercorns, dried rosemary, and garlic cloves. Olives contain 2.8 grams of carbohydrates per 1 cup. Remember to include a small side dish for disposal of the olive pits.

Beef Tenderloin in Red Wine–Peppercorn Sauce

Serves 6
Carb Level: Low

Per serving:

Carbohydrate:	2.3 g
Protein:	42.8 g

Serve with Creamed Spinach (see recipe on page 138).

∾

2 tablespoons olive oil
6 (7-ounce) beef tenderloin
   fillets
Salt and freshly ground black
   pepper to taste
10 ounces beef stock
1 cup dry red wine

2 cloves garlic, pressed
3 tablespoons green peppercorns
$^{1}/_{4}$ cup unsalted butter, cut into
   pieces

1. Heat a large sauté pan on high, and add the oil. Sprinkle the steaks evenly with salt and pepper; place them in the skillet and brown on both sides, about 3 minutes per side. Remove the steaks from the pan, place on a dish, and set aside.

2. Add the beef stock, wine, and garlic to the skillet; cook over high heat for 15 minutes. Return the steaks to the pan and cook for 5 to 6 minutes on each side or to desired doneness. Remove the pan from the heat and remove the steaks, reserving the sauce in the pan. Add the peppercorns and gradually whisk in the butter. Serve the sauce over the steaks.

Safety Tip for Reheating

Re-heated stews and casseroles must be heated to an internal temperature 165° for at least 15 seconds to effectively kill bacteria growth and be considered food safe.

Oysters Rockefeller Soup

2 tablespoons butter

5 celery stalks, finely chopped

2 large onions, finely chopped

1 bay leaf

3 cups chopped fresh spinach

3 cups thinly sliced green onions

1¼ cups chopped fresh flat-leaf parsley

1 clove garlic, minced

1 teaspoon chopped fresh thyme leaves

½ teaspoon crushed dried oregano

2 teaspoons salt

⅛ teaspoon each: freshly ground black pepper, red pepper, and white pepper

1 tablespoon all-purpose flour

30 oysters (about 2 cups)

1 cup chicken stock

¾ cup Pernod (French anise-flavored cordial)

6 cups whipping cream

Serves 12
Carb Level: Moderate

Per serving:	
Carbohydrate:	16.8 g
Protein:	6.7 g

Keep servings to no more than ¾ of a cup each, as this soup is very rich and satisfying.

1. Heat the butter in a Dutch oven over medium-high heat. When the butter starts to foam, add the celery, onion, and bay leaf. Cook for 4 to 5 minutes or until the vegetables are tender. Reduce the heat to low, add the spinach, green onions, and parsley. Cook, stirring constantly, for 3 to 4 minutes. Remove the bay leaf.

2. Add the garlic, thyme, oregano, salt, and peppers. Cook, stirring constantly, for 4 to 5 minutes. Add the flour and cook for 2 minutes, stirring constantly and scraping the sides and bottom of the pan.

3. Drain the oysters, reserving the liquid. Add enough chicken broth to oyster liquid, if necessary, to make 1 cup total; set aside.

4. Increase the heat to medium-high and carefully add the Pernod to the vegetable mixture. Cook, stirring constantly, for 4 to 5 minutes. Add the oyster and stock liquid, and cook for another 3 to 4 minutes. Let cool slightly. Transfer the vegetable mixture to a blender or food processor. Cover and blend or process to a smooth consistency.

5. Return the mixture to the Dutch oven. Stir in whipping cream and cook, over medium heat for 4 to 5 minutes or until heated through, whisking occasionally. Add the oysters and cook for about 5 minutes or until the oyster edges curl. Serve immediately.

Lobster in Vanilla Sauce

Serves 4

Carb Level: Moderate

Per serving:

Carbohydrate:	17.6 g
Protein:	89.0 g

Fish glacé is made by taking 4 ounces of fish stock and simmering it down to 1 ounce.

❧

1 peeled carrot, coarsely chopped
1 large onion, coarsely chopped
1 celery stalk, coarsely chopped
A few parsley stems
1 clove garlic, peeled and
  chopped
4 to 5 black peppercorns
2 bay leaves
Pinch of thyme and tarragon
Salt to taste
2 quarts fish stock or water
1 vanilla bean, sliced in half
  lengthwise
2 quarts dry white wine
4 lobster tails

Vanilla Sauce:

4 shallots, chopped
1 teaspoon unsalted butter
2 ounces dry white wine
1 vanilla bean
1 quart whipping cream
Fish glacé
Salt and freshly ground black
  pepper to taste

1. To prepare the court bouillon, simmer all the ingredients up to and including the fish stock (*or* water) for 1 hour. Add the vanilla bean and white wine and bring to a boil. Add the lobster tails and boil for 8 to 10 minutes, until cooked. Remove the tails. When the lobsters have cooled, remove the meat from the tails and slice into medallions and reserve.

2. To prepare the vanilla sauce, briefly sauté the shallots in the butter in a large sauté pan over medium-high heat. Add the white wine and the vanilla bean. (Split the bean in half lengthwise and scoop out pulp with a small knife to ensure the most efficient use of the vanilla bean. The black specks are the vanilla bean trademark and hold all the flavor). Simmer until almost dry. Add the cream and the fish glacé. Bring to a boil. Reduce the heat and simmer for about 5 minutes. Add salt and pepper to taste. Arrange the lobster meat on individual serving plates and top with the sauce.

Glazed Carrots
with Balsamic Vinegar

3½ pounds baby carrots or
    regular carrots
½ cup butter
6 tablespoons sugar
⅓ cup balsamic vinegar

Salt and freshly ground black
    pepper to taste
¼ cup chopped fresh chives
    for garnish

1. Peel the carrots and cut into 2-inch pieces, halved lengthwise.
2. Melt the butter in a large sauté pan over medium heat. Add the carrots and cook them for about 5 minutes. Cover and cook for another 7 minutes or until slightly tender. Stir in the sugar and vinegar; cook, uncovered, until the carrots are tender and glazed and the liquid has reduced. Season with salt and pepper.
3. Serve in a warm bowl and garnish with fresh chives.

Serves 10
Carb Level: Moderate
Per serving:

Carbohydrate:	18.6 g
Protein:	1.4 g

A colorful and flavorful side for a holiday meal.

❧

Glazed Baked Ham with Rosemary

4-pound boneless ham
30 whole cloves
3 tablespoons Major Grey's Chutney
1 packed tablespoon dark
    brown sugar

2 tablespoons prepared horse-
    radish mustard
2 teaspoons fresh rosemary
    leaves

1. Preheat the oven to 325°.
2. Place the ham in a roasting pan set on a rack. Insert the whole cloves all over the ham, and bake for about 1½ hours or until the internal temperature reads 130°.
3. Meanwhile, in a small saucepan combine the chutney, brown sugar, mustard, and rosemary. Cook over low heat until warm and liquefied. Drizzle the sauce all over the ham and bake for an additional 30 minutes or until the internal temperature reads 140°. The outside of the ham should be crusty and sugary brown.

Serves 12
Carb Level: Moderate
Per serving:

Carbohydrate:	20.0 g
Protein:	27.6 g

This ham tastes great served either hot or cold. Serve it the next day as sandwiches.

❧

Butternut Squash and Turnip Gratin with Gruyère

2 pounds butternut squash

3 large turnips

1 teaspoon chopped fresh thyme

1 teaspoon chopped fresh marjoram

1 teaspoon chopped fresh sage

Salt and freshly ground black pepper to taste

3 garlic cloves, peeled and minced

2 cups heavy cream

4 ounces Gruyère cheese, grated

1. Preheat oven to 375°. Butter a 9" × 12" gratin dish.
2. Peel the squash and trim off the tops and bottoms. Cut off the seed-filled bottom halves, cut it in half lengthwise, and scoop out the seeds. Slice the necks of the squash into $1/8$-inch rounds and slice the base into $1/8$-inch half circles.
3. Peel the turnips and cut them in half lengthwise. Cut them into $1/8$-inch half moons.
4. In a small bowl, combine the thyme, marjoram, and sage.
5. Beginning with the half circles of squash, layer about $1/3$ of the squash slices into the gratin dish. Sprinkle with some of the herbs and season with salt and pepper. Layer the turnip slices over the squash layer. Sprinkle with some of the herbs and half of the minced garlic. Season with salt and pepper.
6. Spread another $1/3$ of the squash slices on top of the turnips. Sprinkle with some herbs and season with salt and pepper. Spread the remaining turnips in another layer over the squash. Sprinkle with some herbs and the rest of the garlic. Top with the remaining squash and herbs, and season with salt and pepper.
7. Slowly pour the cream over the top and down the sides of the dish. Add enough to just barely cover the vegetables when pressed down.
8. Cover the dish with foil. Place the dish on a baking sheet in case any cream bubbles over the edges. Bake for about 45 minutes. Remove the foil and sprinkle with the cheese. Continue to bake, uncovered, for about 25 minutes or until the cheese is lightly browned. Allow to rest for 10 minutes before cutting into it.

Fennel- and Garlic-Crusted Pork Roast

1 small head fennel, coarsely
   chopped
½ cup coarsely chopped onion
2 tablespoons olive oil
6 cloves garlic, peeled and
   sliced

¼ cup chopped fresh assorted
   herbs (thyme, sage, rosemary, parsley, oregano, etc.)
2 teaspoons fennel seeds
Freshly ground black pepper
4½-pound pork rib roast, tied
Salt

Serves 6
Carb Level: Low

Per serving:

Carbohydrate:	5.5 g
Protein:	58.8 g

Your butcher will pre-
pare and tie your rib
roast for roasting.

∾

1. In a blender or food processor, combine the fennel, onion, olive oil, and garlic; purée into a paste. Add the herbs, fennel seeds, and pepper; pulse to combine.
2. With a small sharp knife, make shallow diamond cuts into the skin of the pork roast. Season it all over with salt, rubbing it in well. Rub the garlic-fennel paste over the roast to cover it with a layer about ¼-inch thick. Cover and refrigerate for up to 8 hours. Remove from the refrigerator and let stand at room temperature for about 20 minutes.
3. Preheat the oven to 375°.
4. Transfer the roast to a roasting pan with a rack. Roast for about 1 hour and 15 minutes or until the internal temperature reads 150°. Remove the roast from the oven and allow to rest for at least 20 minutes. Slice the roast into thick chops.

What Is Fennel?

Fennel is a broad bulblike vegetable cultivated in the Mediterranean and the United States. It has long been believed in many cultures to have medicinal qualities. Both the base and stems can be eaten raw as a flavorful addition to salads. Fennel can be cooked in a variety of ways, including braising, grilling, roasting, and sautéing. Fennel is often mislabeled as "sweet anise." The flavor of fennel is much lighter and sweeter than licorice-tasting anise. Fennel contains 4.3 grams of carbohydrates per ¼ cup.

Spicy Chilled Shrimp

Serves 12

Carb Level: Low

Per serving:

Carbohydrate:	5.7 g
Protein:	23.7 g

Keep the shrimp chilled and put the serving bowl on ice while serving.

❧

3 pounds, uncooked shrimp, tail on, peeled and deveined
¾ cup olive oil
½ cup chopped fresh cilantro
¼ cup white wine vinegar
3 tablespoons fresh lemon juice
3 jalapeño chilies, seeded, minced
3 large cloves garlic, minced
¼ teaspoon cayenne pepper
Salt and freshly ground black pepper to taste
3 large lemons, sliced
1 large red onion, sliced

1. Boil the shrimp until pink and opaque, about 3 minutes. When done, chill shrimp in ice water; drain; put in the refrigerator.
2. Whisk next 8 ingredients. Pour the remaining marinade over the shrimp; toss to coat. Layer the shrimp, lemon slices, and onion in a large glass bowl. Cover and refrigerate for 4 hours.

Egg Salad with Endive Leaves

Serves 6

Carb Level: Low

Per serving:

Carbohydrate:	5.1 g
Protein:	10.1 g

Fan the endive spears in a star pattern around the egg salad for a festive presentation.

❧

6 tablespoons mayonnaise
1 tablespoon Dijon mustard
8 hard-boiled eggs, peeled and chopped
¼ cup finely chopped onion
¼ cup finely chopped celery stalks
¼ cup chopped fresh parsley
Salt and white pepper to taste
24 Belgian endive spears, separated
Paprika for garnish

Mix the mayonnaise and mustard in a medium-size bowl. Add the chopped eggs, onion, celery, and parsley. Season with salt and pepper. Cover the egg salad with plastic wrap and refrigerate until ready to serve. Place the egg salad in serving bowl on a platter surrounded with the endive spears. Dust with paprika for color.

Chili Cheese Corn Casserole

4 cups fresh corn kernels, or
   frozen, thawed and drained
1 cup grated Cheddar cheese
1 (8-ounce) package cream
   cheese, at room temperature

1 (7-ounce) can diced green
   chilies
2 teaspoons chili powder
2 teaspoons ground cumin

1. Preheat oven to 350°. Butter a 1½-quart baking dish.
2. Mix all the ingredients in a large bowl until well blended. Transfer to
   the prepared baking dish; bake until bubbling, about 30 minutes. Let
   cool, then cover and refrigerate up to 1 day. To serve, gently reheat,
   covered, in a 350° oven for about 30 minutes until heated throughout.

Serves 8
Carb Level: Moderate

Per serving:

Carbohydrate:	17.9 g
Protein:	8.7 g

An easy dish to pre-
pare the day before
an outdoor picnic.

ᔕ

Spicy Cucumber Relish

2 seedless cucumbers
2 medium shallots, peeled and
   trimmed
1½ tablespoons minced jalapeño
   pepper
1½ loosely packed cups fresh
   mint, chopped medium-fine

2 tablespoons white wine vinegar
   or champagne vinegar
1 teaspoon salt
¼ teaspoon freshly ground black
   pepper
3 tablespoons olive oil

1. Peel the cucumbers. Cut in half lengthwise, remove any seeds, and cut
   crosswise into ⅛-inch slices.
2. Combine the cucumbers, shallots, jalapeño, and mint. In a small bowl,
   combine the vinegar, salt, and pepper. Gradually whisk in the olive oil
   until combined. Pour over the cucumbers, and toss gently to combine.
   Serve.

Serves 10
Carb Level: Low

Per serving:

Carbohydrate:	4.7 g
Protein:	1.2 g

Smaller cucumbers
have fewer seeds than
larger ones.

ᔕ

Tandoori Chicken Kebabs

Serves 8
Carb Level: Low

Per serving:

Carbohydrate:	7.1 g
Protein:	24.5 g

The creamy yogurt sauce offsets the heat of the spices on the chicken.

℘

2 cups plain low-fat yogurt
½ cup chopped fresh cilantro
¼ cup fresh lemon juice
2 tablespoons peeled and grated fresh ginger
2 large cloves garlic, minced
4 teaspoons paprika
2 teaspoons curry powder
1 teaspoon ground cumin
1 teaspoon ground coriander
½ teaspoon cayenne pepper

2 pounds boneless, skinless chicken breasts, cut into 1-inch cubes
4 medium-size red bell peppers, cut into 1-inch pieces
16 bamboo skewers, soaked in water for 30 minutes

1. Purée the first 10 ingredients in a blender or food processor. Pour ½ cup of the mixture into a small bowl, cover, and chill. Pour the remaining mixture into a large bowl, add the chicken, and toss to coat. Cover and chill for at least 1 hour or up to 24 hours.
2. Preheat a gas or charcoal grill or grill pan to medium-high heat. Make sure the grill grate is clean and lightly oiled to prevent sticking.
3. Thread the red bell peppers and chicken on skewers. Grill the kebabs until the chicken is cooked through, about 7 minutes per side. Serve with the reserved yogurt mixture for dipping.

Grilled Beef and Onion Kebabs

4 teaspoons finely ground
   whole coriander seeds
4 teaspoons finely ground
   anise seeds
1 tablespoon minced garlic
1 tablespoon ground paprika
¼ teaspoon cayenne pepper
½ cup olive oil, divided

Salt and freshly ground black
   pepper to taste
1½ pounds boneless sirloin
   steak, fat trimmed, cut into
   1¼-inch cubes
12 red pearl onions (about
   3 ounces), peeled and cut
   in half lengthwise

Serves 4	
Carb Level: Low	
Per serving:	
Carbohydrate:	5.0 g
Protein:	13.1 g

An easy summer recipe that will please everyone!

∽

1. Preheat a grill or grill pan until hot.
2. Place the ground coriander and anise seeds in a medium-size bowl. Add the garlic, paprika, cayenne pepper, and ¼ cup olive oil. Season the marinade with salt and pepper, and stir until combined. Add the sirloin cubes, and stir to coat; set aside.
3. In a medium-size bowl, combine the onions and the remaining olive oil. Season with salt and pepper; toss to coat.
4. Divide the steaks among 4 skewers; thread, leaving ½ inch between each cube. Divide the onions among another 4 skewers; thread.
5. Grill the sirloin kebobs until well browned and medium-rare, and grill the onion until glistening, tender, and slightly charred, 5 to 7 minutes for both. Serve on the skewers.

Summer Skewer Fun

Try some unusual twists on skewers: Fruit skewers—Use colorful bites of strawberries, grapes, and melon pieces. Greek island skewers—Petite pieces of Feta cheese skewered with broiled cherry tomatoes (count 1 gram of carbohydrate per cherry tomato) and pitted Kalamata olives. This is an attractive presentation with fresh rosemary branches for the skewers. Trim the base end of the branch to a point and remove a portion of the rosemary needles, leaving the top of the branch intact.

APPENDIX A
Easy Dishes at a Glance

❖ ❖ ❖

Artichoke Bottoms with Herbed Cheese / 7

Artichoke, Cucumber, and Tomato Salad / 245

Asian-Style Paste / 12

Avocado and Cucumber Salad in Mint Dressing / 96

Avocado and Tomato Dip / 267

Avocado with Tuna Salad / 164

Bacon, Lettuce, Tomato, and Cheese Salad / 174

Baked Garlic Tomatoes / 147

Balsamic-Marinated Beef Tenderloin / 24

Balsamic Vinaigrette / 110

Barbecued Beef / 235

Basic Party Dip and Five Variations / 14

Beef Provençal / 49

Beet Dip / 290

Blanc Manger / 212

Blue Cheese Dressing / 109

Braised Baby Bok Choy / 142

Braised Brisket / 286

Braised Savoy Cabbage / 145

Broccoli Bacon Salad / 162

Broiled Marinated Steak-Bistecca / 65

Caponata / 8

Caprese Salad / 104

Caribbean Shrimp Stew / 114

Cauliflower Vichyssoise / 238

Celery Root and Pear Purée / 289

Champagne-Marinated Summer Berries / 206

Chicken, Blue Cheese, and Apple Salad / 97

Chicken Breast Paillards Layered with Proscuitto and Cheese / 62

Chicken Grape Salad / 155

Chicken with Nectarine Salsa / 275

Chili Cheese Corn Casserole / 299

Chipotle Shrimp / 20

Chocolate Fudge / 209

Chopped Liver / 288

Chutney-Glazed Smoked Ham / 225

Classic Coleslaw / 137

Classic Gazpacho / 73

Coconut Chicken / 86

Cold Fennel Soup / 126

Collard Greens / 137

Coriander Crusted Flank Steak / 232

Corn and Egg Pudding / 201

Cornbread Stuffing / 283

Crabmeat on Red Pepper Strips / 3

Crab Salad / 268

Cream Cheese and Scallion Scramble / 193

Creamed Spinach / 138

Creamy Garlic and Fennel Soup / 21

Creamy Horseradish Dressing / 110

Crêpes / 35

Curried Chicken Spread / 163

Denver Scramble / 199

Deviled Eggs / 178

Drunken Chicken / 75

Egg Custard / 209

Egg Salad with Endive Leaves / 298

Eggplant Topped with Gruyère Cheese / 266

Fennel, Mushroom, and Parmesan Salad / 101

Fiesta Salsa / 74

Fresh Mozzarella Salad / 172

Fried Green Tomatoes / 243

Garlic-Ginger Brussels Sprouts / 148

Garlic Shrimp with Salsa / 74

Glazed Carrots with Balsamic Vinegar / 295

Greek Chicken Lemon Soup / 119

Greek Salad / 100

Green Beans with Shallots and Rosemary / 269

Grilled Beef with Onion Kebabs / 301

Grilled Lamb Chops with Provençal Roasted Tomatoes / 44

Grilled Mushrooms and Peppers / 231

Grilled Pineapple and Avocado Chutney / 9

Grilled Radicchio / 277

Grilled Red Snapper with Basil Aioli / 223

Grilled Spicy Chicken Salad / 152

Grilled Tomatoes / 277

Grilled Zucchini with Balsamic Vinegar / 132

Guacamole / 77

Halibut Ceviche with Herbs / 72

Ham and Cheese Salad / 107

Ham Cornets / 5

Hard-Boiled Egg Salad / 153

Hearts of Romaine with Parmesan Dressing / 176

Hearty Mushroom Soup / 125

Hollandaise Sauce / 192

Homemade Pickles / 133

Hot Artichoke Dip / 3

Jalapeño Paste / 12

Jicama and Chorizo Chips / 2

Layered Taco Salad / 170

Lemon-Spiked Pineapple Smoothie / 31

Lime-Broiled Catfish / 179

Marinated Beefsteak Tomatoes / 141

Mesclun and Fresh Herb Salad / 104

Mexican-Style Shrimp Cocktail / 261

Mexican Tomato Salad / 78

Mock Caviar / 10

Mushroom Curry Sauté / 171

Mushrooms Au Gratin / 264

Mushrooms with Mediterranean Stuffing / 4

Mussels Steamed in White Wine / 254

New Orleans Muffuletta Salad / 165

Olive Tapanade / 10

Onion Soup with Sherry / 121

Orange-Cucumber Salsa / 262

Orange Vinaigrette / 111

Oven-Roasted Winter Vegetables / 280

Parmesan Crisps / 7

Party Cheese Balls / 2

Pear and Pumpkin Soup / 281

Pecan Crusted Catfish with Wilted Greens / 252

Peppered Swordfish / 22

Pesto-Baked Chicken / 226

Pineapple-Ginger Smoothie / 32

Pompano with Salsa Fresca / 76

Pork and Veal Pâté / 34

Pork Roast / 227

Portobellos Stuffed with Basil and Salmon on Arugula Leaves / 54

Pulled Chicken Salad / 153

Ranch Dressing / 109

Rapini with Chili Sauce / 130

Red Cabbage Soup / 128

Red Onions Braised with Sherry Vinegar / 143

Red Snapper with Cayenne Tomato Sauce / 42

Roasted Grouper with Tomatoes / 247

Roasted Pork with Asian Glaze / 80

Roasted Vidalia Onions / 228

Salmon Fillets with Basil / 272

Sausage Appetizers / 13

Sautéed Brussels Sprouts with Butter and Pecans / 136

Sautéed Green Beans with Shiitake Mushrooms / 282

Sautéed Mushrooms with Tarragon / 143

Sautéed Sausage and Peppers / 156

Sautéed Spinach with Pine Nuts / 276

Scrambled Eggs with Lox and Onions / 197

Seared Salmon Carpaccio / 218

Sherry Vinaigrette / 111

Shrimp Salad / 164

Shrimp Scampi / 271

Shrimp with Plum Dipping Sauce / 82

Sicilian-Style Tomatoes / 131

Smoked Salmon Rillette / 219

Smoked Shrimp with Horseradish Cream / 258

Smoked Trout and Watercress Salad / 27

Smoked Whitefish Salad / 285

Soy Sauce Vinaigrette / 112

Spanish Marinated Olives / 257

Spanish Stuffed Veal Chops / 28

Spiced Carrots / 147

Spicy Chicken Wings / 184

Spicy Chilled Shrimp / 298

Spicy Cucumber Relish / 299

Spicy Jicama Chips / 5

Spicy Olive and Walnut Tapenade / 268

Spicy Pork Roast / 71

Spinach and Ricotta Dip / 4

Spinach and Ricotta Filling / 219

Spinach, Bacon, and Goat Cheese Salad / 98

Spinach Salad with Warm Bacon Dressing / 175

Steamed Clams with Cilantro-Garlic Essence / 19

Stewed Pepper and Tomato Purée / 265

Strawberry Jam / 192

Stuffed Tomato with Cottage Cheese / 157

Tandoori Chicken Kebabs / 300

Teriyaki Beef / 158

Thai Beef Salad / 92

Thai Vinaigrette / 91

Tomato Bisque / 119

Tomato Sauce / 67

Tomatoes with Green Goddess Dressing / 103

Trout Grenobloise / 50

Tuna Steaks with Wasabi-Coconut Sauce / 29

Tuna Tapenade / 271

Turkey Meatballs with Tomato Sauce / 291

Tuscan Lamb Chops / 63

Vegetable Cottage Cheese Spread / 163

Vegetable Egg Salad / 162

Venetian Liver and Onions / 58

Warm Berry Compote / 206

Warm Spinach and Artichoke Dip / 16

White Wine–Poached Salmon / 224

Zucchini Frittata / 200

❖ ❖ ❖

Index

A

Additives, 186
Ahi tuna steaks, 30
Antipasto, 56
Appetizers
  Artichoke Bottoms with Herbed
    Cheese, 7
  Asian-Style Paste, 12
  Basic Party Dip and Variations, 14–15
  Caponata, 8
  Crabmeat on Red Pepper Strips, 3
  Grilled Pineapple and Avocado
    Chutney, 9
  Ham Cornets, 5
  Hot Artichoke Dip, 3
  Jalapeño Paste, 12
  Jicama and Chorizo Chips, 2
  Mock Caviar, 10
  Mushrooms with Mediterranean
    Stuffing, 4
  Olive Tapenade, 10
  Parmesan Crisps, 7
  Party Cheese Balls, 2
  Pesto Eggplant Caviar, 11
  Portobello Mushrooms with Warm
    Garlic Flan, 6
  Sausage Appetizers, 13
  Spicy Jicama Chips, 5
  Spinach and Ricotta Dip, 4
  Warm Spinach and Artichoke Dip, 16
Artichoke Bottoms with Herbed Cheese, 7
Artichoke, Cucumber, and Tomato Salad,
  245
Arugula, 54
Asian Broccoli, 85
Asian Salmon, 18
Asian Slaw, 93
Asian-Style Paste, 12
Asparagus with Orange Herb Butter, 145
Avocado and Cucumber Salad in Mint
  Dressing, 96
Avocado and Tomato Dip, 267
Avocado with Tuna Salad, 164
Avocados, 96

B

Baby Back Ribs with Sauerkraut, 181
Bacon, Lettuce, and Tomatoes (BLTs),
  178

Bacon, Lettuce, Tomato, and Cheese
  Salad, 174
Baked Cod with Tomatoes, Capers, and
  Sautéed Spinach, 244
Baked Garlic Tomatoes, 147
Baked Haddock with Parsley and
  Lemon, 46
Baked Ocean Perch with Black Olives
  and Capers, 61
Baked Pork Chops with Caramelized
  Onions and Smoked Cheddar, 185
Balsamic-Marinated Beef Tenderloin, 24
Balsamic Vinaigrette, 110
Balsamic vinegar, 228
Barbecued Beef, 235
Basic Party Dip and Five Variations,
  14–15
Beef
  Balsamic-Marinated Beef Tenderloin,
    24
  Barbecued Beef, 235
  Beef Provençal, 49
  Beef Roulade, 166–67
  Beef Salad with Horseradish Dressing,
    173
  Beef Tenderloin in Red
    Wine–Peppercorn Sauce, 292
  Beef Tenderloin with Belgian Endive,
    239
  Beef with Cucumber, 274
  Braised Brisket, 286
  Broiled Marinated Steak-Bistecca, 65
  Classic Meat Loaf, 188
  Corned Beef "Hash", 196
  Grilled Beef and Onion Kebabs, 301
  Grilled Beef Tenderloin with Shiitake
    Sauce, 87
  Herb-Stuffed Flank Steak, 168
  Marinated Grilled Steak Strips, 250
  Pot Roast with Vegetable Sauce, 187
  Steak and Eggs, 194
  Teriyaki Beef, 158
  Thai Beef Salad, 92
  Venetian Liver and Onions, 58
Beet Dip, 290
Berries, carbohydrates in, 32
Berry Treat, 215
Blanc Manger, 212
BLTs, 178
Blue Cheese Dip, 14
Blue Cheese Dressing, 109

Boneless Chicken Thighs with Major
  Grey's Chutney, 233
Bouillabaisse, 115
Bouquet garni, 128
Braised Baby Bok Choy, 142
Braised Brisket, 286
Braised Dover Sole with Béchamel and
  Vegetables, 38–39
Braised Fennel, 140
Braised Savoy Cabbage, 145
Breakfasts, 191–202
Broccoli Bacon Salad, 162
Broiled Marinated Steak-Bistecca, 65
Broiled Scallops with Apple-Wood
  Smoked Bacon, 56
Broiling, 251
Broths, 122
Brussels sprouts, carbohydrates in, 28
Butter, clarified, 42
Butter, storing, 20, 64
Butter, sweet, 42
Butter, unsalted, 20
Butternut Squash and Turnip Gratin with
  Gruyère, 296

C

Caesar Salad with Shrimp, 106
Caffeine, avoiding, 285
Capers, 22, 61
Caponata, 8
Caprese Salad, 104
Carbohydrates, description of, v–vi
Caribbean Shrimp Stew, 114
Cauliflower, as potato substitute, 116, 188
Cauliflower Vichyssoise, 238
Celery Root and Pear Purée, 289
Chafing dish, 269
Champagne-Marinated Summer Berries,
  206
Cheese and Salami Tray, 230
Cheese board, 290
Cheese platters, 252
Cheeses, carbohydrates in, 100
Cheeses, Mexican, 75
Cheeses, Parmesan, 102
Chicken. See Poultry
Chicken and Mushroom Soup, 117
Chicken, Blue Cheese, and Apple Salad,
  97

Chicken Breast Paillards Layered with Prosciutto and Cheese, 62
Chicken Breasts Chasseur, 41
Chicken Cacciatore, 60
Chicken, cooking safely, 275
Chicken Grape Salad, 155
Chicken Pâté, 270
Chicken Potpie Stew, 189
Chicken Skewers with Spicy Island Marinade, 88
Chicken Wings, 257
Chicken with Nectarine Salsa, 275
Chickens Stuffed with Chorizo and Spinach, 70
Chili Cheese Corn Casserole, 299
Chili, experimenting with, 189
Chilies, 76, 77
Chipotle chilies, 76
Chipotle Shrimp, 20
Chocolate-Covered Nuts, 212
Chocolate Fudge, 209
Chocolate Grand Marnier Mousse, 207
Chocolate Meringue Cookies, 208
Chopped Liver, 288
Christmas dishes, 295–97
Chutney-Glazed Smoked Ham, 225
Citrus juice, carbohydrates in, 72, 199
Clams, cooking, 19
Clams, preparing, 121
Clams, purchasing, 19
Classic Coleslaw, 137
Classic Gazpacho, 73
Classic Meat Loaf, 188
Coconut Chicken, 86
Cod Cakes, 230
Cod with Lemongrass Sauce, 90
Coffee, avoiding, 285
Coffee, serving, 221
Cold Fennel Soup, 126
Collard Greens, 137
Comfort foods, 177–89
Cooking techniques, changing, 142
Coriander-Crusted Flank Steak, 232
Corn and Egg Pudding, 201
Cornbread Stuffing, 283
Corned Beef "Hash", 196
Crab Cakes with Red Pepper Sauce, 160–61
Crab Salad, 268
Crabmeat, 268
Crabmeat Omelet, 202

Crabmeat on Red Pepper Strips, 3
Cream Cheese and Scallion Scramble, 193
Cream of Cauliflower Soup, 116
Creamed Spinach, 138
Creamy Garlic and Fennel Soup, 21
Creamy Horseradish Dressing, 110
Creamy Onion Dip, 15
Crêpe Fillings, 36–37
Crêpes, 35–37
Crustless Salmon Potpie, 183
Curried Chicken Chowder, 154–55
Curried Chicken Spread, 163

D

Denver Scramble, 199
Desserts
    Berry Treat, 215
    Blanc Manger, 212
    Champagne-Marinated Summer Berries, 206
    Chocolate-Covered Nuts, 212
    Chocolate Fudge, 209
    Chocolate Grand Marnier Mousse, 207
    Chocolate Meringue Cookies, 208
    Egg Custard, 209
    European-style desserts, 208
    Glazed Bananas, 204
    Mocha Mousse, 214
    No-Crust Cheesecake, 213
    Orange Cups with Lemon Cream, 205
    Pear Dessert Dish, 207
    Refrigerator Pumpkin Pike with Macadamia Nut Crust, 210
    Rhubarb and Strawberry Cream, 215
    Strawberry Treat, 215
    Vanilla Ice Cream, 211
    Warm Berry Compote, 206
    on the Web, 205
Deviled Eggs, 178
Dietary fiber, 281
Dill Dip, 14
Dips
    Avocado and Tomato Dip, 267
    Beet Dip, 290
    Blue Cheese Dip, 14
    Creamy Onion Dip, 15
    Dill Dip, 14
    Guacamole, 77
    Hot Artichoke Dip, 3

Picante Dip, 15
Seafood Dip, 15
Spicy Olive and Walnut Tapenade, 268
Spinach and Ricotta Dip, 4
Tuna Tapenade, 271
Warm Spinach and Artichoke Dip, 16
Dressings. *See also* Salads
    adding, 105
    Balsamic Vinaigrette, 110
    Blue Cheese Dressing, 109
    Creamy Horseradish Dressing, 110
    Green Goddess Dressing, 103
    Lemon Juice, 106
    Mayonnaise Dressing, 108
    Mint Dressing, 96
    Olive Oil Dressing, 98
    Orange Vinaigrette, 111
    Parmesan Dressing, 176
    Ranch Dressing, 109
    Sherry Vinaigrette, 111
    Soy Sauce Vinaigrette, 112
    Warm Bacon Dressing, 175
Drunken Chicken, 75

E

Easy dishes, 302–3
Egg Custard, 209
Egg Salad with Endive Leaves, 298
Eggplant Stew, 123
Eggplant Timbale, 139
Eggplant Topped with Gruyère Cheese, 266
Eggs
    carbohydrates in, 200
    Corn and Egg Pudding, 201
    Crabmeat Omelet, 202
    cracking tip, 214
    Cream Cheese and Scallion Scramble, 193
    Denver Scramble, 199
    Deviled Eggs, 178
    eating raw, 106, 194
    Egg Custard, 209
    Egg Salad with Endive Leaves, 298
    Hard-Boiled Egg Salad, 153
    Hard-Boiled Eggs Stuffed with Mushrooms and Cheese, 259
    Herbed Omelet, 198

Scrambled Eggs with Lox and Onions, 197
shells of, 193
Steak and Eggs, 194
Vegetable Egg Salad, 162
Zucchini Frittata, 200
Entertaining, 255–77

F

Fasting, 274
Fennel, 297
Fennel- and Garlic-Crusted Pork Roast, 297
Fennel, Mushroom, and Parmesan Salad, 101
Fiesta Salsa, 74
Fish. *See* Seafood
Fish, cooking times, 180
Fish, purchasing, 183
Fish Stew, 240
Flowers, food safe, 245
Food safety tips, 13, 106, 126, 194, 233, 275, 292
Fourth of July dishes, 298–301
French entrées
  Baked Haddock with Parsley and Lemon, 46
  Beef Provençal, 49
  Braised Dover Sole with Béchamel and Vegetables, 38–39
  Chicken Breasts Chasseur, 41
  Crepe Fillings, 36–37
  Crepes, 35–37
  Grilled Lamb Chops with Provençal Roasted Tomatoes, 44–45
  Halibut with Porcinis, Shallots, and Tomatoes, 47
  Lemon Chicken, 48
  Mustard-Glazed Monkfish Wrapped in Bacon, 40
  Pork and Veal Pâté, 34
  Red Snapper with Cayenne Tomato Sauce, 42
  Roasted Duck with Lemon, 43
  Trout Grenobloise, 50
  Veal Stew Blanquette, 51
Fresh Mozzarella Salad, 172
Fried Chicken, 182
Fried Green Tomatoes, 243
Fruit, carbohydrates in, 157, 165

Fruit Platter, 230
Fruit, purchasing, 27

G

Garlic-Ginger Brussels Sprouts, 148
Garlic, purchasing, 21
Garlic, roasting, 246, 289
Garlic Shrimp with Salsa, 74
Ginger, storing, 92
Glazed Baked Ham with Rosemary, 295
Glazed Bananas, 204
Glazed Carrots with Balsamic Vinegar, 295
Greek Chicken Lemon Soup, 119
Greek Salad, 100
Green Beans with Shallots and Rosemary, 269
Green Goddess Dressing, 103
Grilled Beef and Onion Kebabs, 301
Grilled Beef Tenderloin with Shiitake Sauce, 87
Grilled Lamb Chops with Provençal Roasted Tomatoes, 44–45
Grilled Lobster with Lemon and Tarragon, 220
Grilled Mediterranean Grouper, 237
Grilled Mushrooms and Peppers, 231
Grilled Pineapple and Avocado Chutney, 9
Grilled Radicchio, 277
Grilled Radicchio with Fontina Cheese, 138
Grilled Red Snapper with Basil Aioli, 223
Grilled Spicy Chicken Salad, 152
Grilled Swordfish with Olive Tapenade, 251
Grilled Swordfish with Wasabi and Spinach, 81
Grilled Tomatoes, 277
Grilled Tuna with Asian Slaw, 93
Grilled Zucchini with Balsamic Vinegar, 132
Grilling, 251
Guacamole, 77

H

Halibut Ceviche with Herbs, 72
Halibut with Porcinis, Shallots, and Tomatoes, 47

Ham and Cheese Salad, 107
Ham Cornets, 5
Hanukkah dishes, 285–88
Hard-Boiled Egg Salad, 153
Hard-Boiled Eggs Stuffed with Mushrooms and Cheese, 259
Hearts of Romaine with Parmesan Dressing, 176
Hearty Mushroom Soup, 125
Herb Chicken Stew, 124
Herb-Stuffed Flank Steak, 168
Herbed Omelet, 198
Herbs, 59, 128, 198
Holiday dishes, 279–301
Hollandaise Sauce, 192
Homemade Breakfast Sausage Patties, 195
Homemade Pickles, 133
Hot Artichoke Dip, 3

I

Italian dishes
  Baked Ocean Perch with Black Olives and Capers, 61
  Broiled Marinated Steak-Bistecca, 65
  Broiled Scallops with Apple-Wood Smoked Bacon, 56
  Chicken Breast Paillards Layered with Prosciutto and Cheese, 62
  Chicken Cacciatore, 60
  Pork Chops Braised in White Wine, 66
  Portobellos Stuffed with Basil and Salmon on Arugula Leaves, 54
  Rabbit and Herb Stew, 59
  Tuscan Lamb Chops, 63
  Veal Cutlets with Ricotta Cheese and Spinach, 55
  Veal Osso Buco, 57
  Veal Scallops with Marsala Wine, 64
  Venetian Liver and Onions, 58

J, L

Jalapeño Paste, 12
Jalapeños, 76
Jell-O, 182
Jicama, 78
Jicama and Chorizo Chips, 2
Juices, carbohydrates in, 72, 199

Lamb
    Grilled Lamb Chops with Provençal
        Roasted Tomatoes, 44–45
    Lamb Stew with Herbs de Provence,
        127
    Spring Lamb Chops, 221
    Tuscan Lamb Chops, 63
Latkes, 184
Layered Taco Salad, 170
Lemon Chicken, 48
Lemon Chicken Drumettes, 256–57
Lemon-Spiked Pineapple Smoothie, 31
Lime-Broiled Catfish, 179
Lobster and Asparagus Salad, 108
Lobster in Vanilla Sauce, 294
Lobster serving tips, 220
Lunches, 151–76

M

Marinated Beefsteak Tomatoes, 141
Marinated Grilled Steak Strips, 250
Matzo Ball Soup, 287
Medications and vitamins, 197
Mesclun and Fresh Herb Salad, 104
Mexican cheeses, 75
Mexican green tomato, 262
Mexican potato, 78
Mexican specialties
    Chickens Stuffed with Chorizo and
        Spinach, 70
    Classic Gazpacho, 73
    Drunken Chicken, 75
    Fiesta Salsa, 74
    Garlic Shrimp with Salsa, 74
    Halibut Ceviche with Herbs, 72
    Mexican-Style Shrimp Cocktail, 261
    Mexican Tomato Salad, 78
    Pompano with Salsa Fresca, 76
    Salsas, 74
    Spicy Pork Roast, 71
Milk, carbohydrates in, 201
Mint Dressing, 96
Miso, 88
Mocha Mousse, 214
Mock Caviar, 10
Mushroom Curry Sauté, 171
Mushroom Custard with Blood Oranges
    and Crispy Greens, 99
Mushrooms Au Gratin, 264
Mushrooms, rehydrating, 127

Mushrooms with Mediterranean Stuffing,
    4
Mussel Salad with Green Beans, 260
Mussels, preparing, 121
Mussels Steamed in White Wine, 254
Mustard-Glazed Monkfish Wrapped in
    Bacon, 40

N

New Orleans Muffuletta Salad, 165
New Year's Eve dishes, 289–94
No-Crust Cheesecake, 213
Nutritional analyses, vi
Nuts, carbohydrates in, 31

O

Olive oils, 24, 65
Olive Tapenade, 10
Olives, 291
Onion Soup with Sherry, 121
Onions, chopping, 71
Onions, substituting, 86
Orange-Cucumber Salsa, 262
Orange Cups with Lemon Cream, 205
Orange Vinaigrette, 111
Organic foods, 156
Oven-Roasted Winter Vegetables, 280
Oysters Rockefeller Soup, 293

P

Parmesan cheese, 102
Parmesan Crisps, 7
Party Cheese Balls, 2
Pear and Pumpkin Soup, 281
Pear Dessert Dish, 207
Pears Wrapped in Prosciutto, 105
Pecan-Crusted Catfish with Wilted
    Greens, 252
Peppered Swordfish, 22
Pesto-Baked Chicken, 226
Pesto Eggplant Caviar, 11
Picante Dip, 15
Pineapple-Ginger Smoothie, 32
Pompano with Salsa Fresca, 76
Pork
    Baby Back Ribs with Sauerkraut, 181
    Baked Pork Chops with Caramelized
        Onions and Smoked Cheddar, 185
    Chutney-Glazed Smoked Ham, 225

Fennel- and Garlic-Crusted Pork Roast,
    297
Glazed Baked Ham with Rosemary,
    295
Homemade Breakfast Sausage Patties,
    195
Pork and Veal Pâté, 34
Pork Chops Braised in White Wine,
    66
Pork Crown Roast, 229
Pork Roast, 227
Roasted Pork with Asian Glaze, 80
Sautéed Ham with a Cider Reduction,
    234
Sautéed Sausage and Peppers, 156
Spicy Pork Roast, 71
Portobello Mushrooms with Warm Garlic
    Flan, 6
Portobellos Stuffed with Basil and
    Salmon on Arugula Leaves, 54
Pot Roast with Vegetable Sauce, 187
Potatoes, substituting, 116, 184, 188
Poultry
    Boneless Chicken Thighs with Major
        Grey's Chutney, 233
    Chicken Breast Paillards Layered with
        Prosciutto and Cheese, 62
    Chicken Breasts Chasseur, 41
    Chicken Cacciatore, 60
    Chicken Potpie Stew, 189
    Chicken Skewers with Spicy Island
        Marinade, 88
    Chicken Wings, 257
    Chicken with Nectarine Salsa, 275
    Chickens Stuffed with Chorizo and
        Spinach, 70
    Coconut Chicken, 86
    Drunken Chicken, 75
    Fried Chicken, 182
    Grilled Spicy Chicken Salad, 152
    Lemon Chicken, 48
    Lemon Chicken Drumettes, 256–57
    Pesto-Baked Chicken, 226
    Pulled Chicken Salad, 153
    Roast Pheasant with Cabbage, 222–23
    Roasted Chicken Stuffed with Herbed
        Goat Cheese, 23
    Roasted Duck with Lemon, 43
    Spicy Chicken Wings, 184
    Tandoori Chicken Kebabs, 300

Turkey Meatballs with Tomato Sauce, 291
Protein, 130
Pulled Chicken Salad, 153

R

Rabbit
  Rabbit and Herb Stew, 59
  Roasted Rabbit with Garlic, 246
Ranch Dressing, 109
Rapini with Chili Sauce, 130
Red Cabbage Soup, 128
Red Onions Braised with Sherry Vinegar, 143
Red Snapper with Cayenne Tomato Sauce, 42
Red Snapper with Garlic Ginger Sauce, 83
Refrigerator Pumpkin Pie with Macadamia Nut Crust, 210
Reheating tips, 126, 292
Rhubarb and Strawberry Cream, 215
Roast Pheasant with Cabbage, 222–23
Roasted Beet Salad, 102
Roasted Chicken Stuffed with Herbed Goat Cheese, 23
Roasted Duck with Lemon, 43
Roasted Eggplant Napoleon with Marinated Goat Cheese, 242–43
Roasted Grouper with Tomatoes, 247
Roasted Pork with Asian Glaze, 80
Roasted Rabbit with Garlic, 246
Roasted Salmon with Goat Cheese and Tarragon, 253
Roasted Tomato Onion Soup, 25
Roasted Vidalia Onions, 228
Rosemary Jus, 284

S

Sage- and Pancetta-Wrapped Shrimp, 26
Salads. *See also* Dressings
  adding dressing, 105
  Artichoke, Cucumber, and Tomato Salad, 245
  Avocado and Cucumber Salad in Mint Dressing, 96
  Avocado with Tuna Salad, 164
  Bacon, Lettuce, Tomato, and Cheese Salad, 174
  Beef Salad with Horseradish Dressing, 173
  Broccoli Bacon Salad, 162
  Caesar Salad with Shrimp, 106
  Caprese Salad, 104
  Chicken, Blue Cheese, and Apple Salad, 97
  Chicken Grape Salad, 155
  Crab Salad, 268
  Egg Salad with Endive Leaves, 298
  Fennel, Mushroom, and Parmesan Salad, 101
  Fresh Mozzarella Salad, 172
  garnishes for, 103
  Greek Salad, 100
  Grilled Spicy Chicken Salad, 152
  Ham and Cheese Salad, 107
  Hard-Boiled Egg Salad, 153
  Hearts of Romaine with Parmesan Dressing, 176
  Layered Taco Salad, 170
  Lobster and Asparagus Salad, 108
  Mesclun and Fresh Herb Salad, 104
  Mexican Tomato Salad, 78
  Mushroom Custard with Blood Oranges and Crispy Greens, 99
  Mussel Salad with Green Beans, 260
  New Orleans Muffuletta Salad, 165
  Pears Wrapped in Prosciutto, 105
  Pulled Chicken Salad, 153
  Roasted Beet Salad, 102
  Shrimp Salad, 164
  Smoked Trout and Watercress Salad, 27
  Smoked Whitefish Salad, 285
  Spinach, Bacon, and Goat Cheese Salad, 98
  Spinach Salad with Warm Bacon Dressing, 175
  Thai Beef Salad, 92
  Tomatoes with Green Goddess Dressing, 103
  Vegetable Egg Salad, 162
  washing greens, 107
Salmon Fillets with Basil, 272
Salmon with Chive Mustard Butter, 180
Salmonella, 106, 194
Salsas
  carbohydrates in, 74
  Chicken with Nectarine Salsa, 275
  Fiesta Salsa, 74
  Orange-Cucumber Salsa, 262
  Salsa Cruda, 74
  Salsa Fresca, 76
  Salsa Verde, 74
Salt, types of, 152
Sauces
  Adobo sauce, 76
  Béchamel Sauce, 39
  Brandy and Cream Sauce, 146
  Brown Sauce, 166
  Chili Sauce, 84, 130
  Garlic Ginger Sauce, 83
  Ginger Sauce, 89
  Hollandaise Sauce, 192
  Lemongrass Sauce, 90
  Mustard Dill Sauce, 146
  Plum Dipping Sauce, 82
  Red Pepper Sauce, 160–61
  Rosemary Jus, 284
  Shiitake Sauce, 87
  Soy Sauce, 167
  Stewed Pepper and Tomato Purée, 265
  Thai Vinaigrette, 91
  Tomato Sauce, 42, 67, 291
  Vanilla Sauce, 294
  Vinaigrette, 91
  Wasabi-Coconut Sauce, 29
Sauerkraut, 179
Sausage Appetizers, 13
Sausage, carbohydrates in, 195
Sautéed Brussels Sprouts with Butter and Pecan, 136
Sautéed Green Beans with Shiitake Mushrooms, 282
Sautéed Ham with a Cider Reduction, 234
Sautéed Mushrooms with Tarragon, 143
Sautéed Sausage and Peppers, 156
Sautéed Spinach with Pine Nuts, 276
Sautéed Swordfish in a White Wine Sauce, 236
Sautéed Zucchini with Mustard Dill Sauce, 144
Scallops in an Herbed Tomato Sauce, 273
Scrambled Eggs with Lox and Onions, 197
Sea Scallops with Ginger Sauce, 89
Seafood
  Asian Salmon, 18

Baked Cod with Tomatoes, Capers, and Sautéed Spinach, 244
Baked Haddock with Parsley and Lemon, 46
Baked Ocean Perch with Black Olives and Capers, 61
Braised Dover Sole with Béchamel and Vegetables, 38–39
Broiled Scallops with Apple-Wood Smoked Bacon, 56
Chipotle Shrimp, 20
Cod Cakes, 230
Cod with Lemongrass Sauce, 90
Crab Cakes with Red Pepper Sauce, 160–61
Crabmeat Omelet, 202
Crustless Salmon Potpie, 183
Fish Stew, 240
Garlic Shrimp with Salsa, 74
Grilled Lobster with Lemon and Tarragon, 220
Grilled Mediterranean Grouper, 237
Grilled Red Snapper with Basil Aioli, 223
Grilled Swordfish with Olive Tapenade, 251
Grilled Swordfish with Wasabi and Spinach, 81
Grilled Tuna with Asian Slaw, 93
Halibut Ceviche with Herbs, 72
Halibut with Porcinis, Shallots, and Tomatoes, 47
Lime-Broiled Catfish, 179
Lobster in Vanilla Sauce, 294
Mexican-Style Shrimp Cocktail, 261
Mussels Steamed in White Wine, 254
Mustard-Glazed Monkfish Wrapped in Bacon, 40
Pecan-Crusted Catfish with Wilted Greens, 252
Peppered Swordfish, 22
Pompano with Salsa Fresca, 76
Portobellos Stuffed with Basil and Salmon on Arugula Leaves, 54
Red Snapper with Cayenne Tomato Sauce, 42
Red Snapper with Garlic Ginger Sauce, 83
Roasted Grouper with Tomatoes, 247
Roasted Salmon with Goat Cheese and Tarragon, 253

Sage- and Pancetta-Wrapped Shrimp, 26
Salmon Fillets with Basil, 272
Salmon with Chive Mustard Butter, 180
Sautéed Swordfish in a White Wine Sauce, 236
Scallops in an Herbed Tomato Sauce, 273
Sea Scallops with Ginger Sauce, 89
Seafood Dip, 15
Seared Salmon Carpaccio, 218
Shrimp Salad, 164
Shrimp Scampi, 271
Shrimp with Plum Dipping Sauce, 82
Smoked Salmon Rillette, 219
Smoked Shrimp with Horseradish Cream, 258
Smoked Trout and Watercress Salad, 27
Spicy Chilled Shrimp, 298
Steamed Clams with Cilantro-Garlic Essence, 19
Szechuan Shrimp with Chili Sauce, 84
Trout Grenobloise, 50
Tuna Steaks with Wasabi-Coconut Sauce, 29
White Wine-Poached Salmon, 224
Seared Salmon Carpaccio, 218
Shallots, 34
Shellfish, preparing, 121
Sherry Vinaigrette, 111
Shrimp Salad, 164
Shrimp Scampi, 271
Shrimp sizes, 26
Shrimp with Plum Dipping Sauce, 82
Sicilian-Style Tomatoes, 131
Side dishes
    Asparagus with Orange Herb Butter, 145
    Baked Garlic Tomatoes, 147
    Braised Baby Bok Choy, 142
    Braised Fennel, 140
    Braised Savoy Cabbage, 145
    Classic Coleslaw, 137
    Collard Greens, 137
    Creamed Spinach, 138
    Eggplant Timbale, 139
    Garlic-Ginger Brussels Sprouts, 148
    Grilled Radicchio with Fontina Cheese, 138

    Grilled Zucchini with Balsamic Vinegar, 132
    Homemade Pickles, 133
    Marinated Beefsteak Tomatoes, 141
    Rapini with Chili Sauce, 130
    Red Onions Braised with Sherry Vinegar, 143
    Sautéed Brussels Sprouts with Butter and Pecan, 136
    Sautéed Mushrooms with Tarragon, 143
    Sautéed Zucchini with Mustard Dill Sauce, 144
    Sicilian-Style Tomatoes, 131
    Spiced Carrots, 147
    Spinach-Wrapped Zucchini Flan, 135
    Turnip Gratin with Onion and Thyme, 150
    Vegetable Casserole, 134
    Wild Mushrooms in a Brandy and Cream Sauce, 146
    Zucchini Stuffed with Mushrooms, 149
Skewers, 301
Smoked Salmon Rillette, 219
Smoked Shrimp with Horseradish Cream, 258
Smoked Trout and Watercress Salad, 27
Smoked Whitefish Salad, 285
Soups
    Bouillabaisse, 115
    broths for, 122
    Chicken and Mushroom Soup, 117
    Cold Fennel Soup, 126
    Cream of Cauliflower Soup, 116
    Curried Chicken Chowder, 154–55
    freezing, 125
    Greek Chicken Lemon Soup, 119
    Hearty Mushroom Soup, 125
    Matzo Ball Soup, 287
    Mushroom Curry Sauté, 171
    Onion Soup with Sherry, 121
    Oysters Rockefeller Soup, 293
    Pear and Pumpkin Soup, 281
    Red Cabbage Soup, 128
    reheating, 126
    Roasted Tomato Onion Soup, 25
    Stilton and Cheddar Cheese Soup, 118
    Tomato Bisque, 119
Soy Sauce, 167
Soy Sauce Vinaigrette, 112
Spanish Marinated Olives, 257

Spanish Stuffed Veal Chops, 28
Spiced Carrots, 147
Spicy Chicken Wings, 184
Spicy Chilled Shrimp, 298
Spicy Cucumber Relish, 299
Spicy Jicama Chips, 5
Spicy Olive and Walnut Tapenade, 268
Spicy Pork Roast, 71
Spinach and Mushroom Rolls, 159
Spinach and Ricotta Dip, 4
Spinach and Ricotta Filling, 219
Spinach, Bacon, and Goat Cheese Salad, 98
Spinach Salad with Warm Bacon Dressing, 175
Spinach-Wrapped Zucchini Flan, 135
Spring Lamb Chops, 221
Steak and Eggs, 194
Steamed Clams with Cilantro-Garlic Essence, 19
Stewed Pepper and Tomato Purée, 265
Stews
    benefits of, 124
    Caribbean Shrimp Stew, 114
    Eggplant Stew, 123
    Fish Stew, 240
    freezing, 125
    Herb Chicken Stew, 124
    Lamb Stew with Herbs de Provence, 127
    Rabbit and Herb Stew, 59
    reheating, 292
    Texas Chili, 120
    Veal Stew Blanquette, 51
    Vegetable Curry Stew, 122
Stilton and Cheddar Cheese Soup, 118
Strawberries, carbohydrates in, 32, 215
Strawberry Jam, 192
Strawberry Treat, 215
Stuffed Bell Peppers, 186
Stuffed Cabbage Rolls, 169
Stuffed Tomato with Cottage Cheese, 157
Stuffed Zucchini, 263
Sweet butter, 20
Szechuan Shrimp with Chili Sauce, 84

T

Tandoori Chicken Kebabs, 300
Temptation, avoiding, 204
Teriyaki Beef, 158

Texas Chili, 120
Thai Beef Salad, 92
Thai Vinaigrette, 91
Thanksgiving dishes, 280–84
Thermometers, 13
Tofu, 85
Tomatillo, 262
Tomato Bisque, 119
Tomatoes, carbohydrates in, 67
Tomatoes, choosing, 141
Tomatoes, substituting, 77
Tomatoes with Green Goddess Dressing, 103
Trout Grenobloise, 50
Tuna Steaks with Wasabi-Coconut Sauce, 29
Tuna Tapenade, 271
Turkey Meatballs with Tomato Sauce, 291
Turnip Gratin with Onion and Thyme, 150
Tuscan Lamb Chops, 63

V

Vanilla Ice Cream, 211
Veal
    Pork and Veal Pâté, 34
    Spanish Stuffed Veal Chops, 28
    Veal Cutlets with Ricotta Cheese and Spinach, 55
    Veal Osso Buco, 57
    Veal Saltimboca, 248–49
    Veal Scallops with Marsala Wine, 64
    Veal Stew Blanquette, 51
    Veal Stock, 249
Vegetable Casserole, 134
Vegetable Cottage Cheese Spread, 163
Vegetable Curry Stew, 122
Vegetable Egg Salad, 162
Vegetables, as side dishes, 129–50
Vegetables, carbohydrates in, 139, 140, 148, 150
Vegetables, roasting, 276
Venetian Liver and Onions, 58
Venison Medallions with Cranberry Dijon Chutney, 241
Vinaigrette, 91, 237
Vinegar, balsamic, 228
Vinegar, carbohydrates in, 98
Vitamins, absorbing, 136, 197
Vitamins, losing, 238

W

Warm Berry Compote, 206
Warm Spinach and Artichoke Dip, 16
Water, 136
Weekend meals, 217–54
White Wine-Poached Salmon, 224
Wild Mushrooms in a Brandy and Cream Sauce, 146
Wine and Cheese Fondue, 30
Wine, carbohydrates in, 258
Wine, cooking with, 44
Wine, types of, 82

Z

Zucchini Frittata, 200
Zucchini Stuffed with Mushrooms, 149

THE EVERYTHING LOW-FAT HIGH-FLAVOR COOKBOOK

By Lisa Shaw

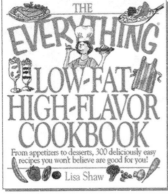

Low-fat cooking is no longer a fad: It has become a way of life for the millions of us who are either battling the bulge or just trying to eat healthy. *The Everything® Low-Fat High-Flavor Cookbook* features over 300 delicious recipes that are easy to prepare and can be created with the ingredients found in any kitchen. The fat-reducing tricks and techniques used in this book have been perfected, so you won't even miss the artery-clogging ingredients you craved in your favorite entrées, salads, and even desserts!

Trade paperback,
$14.95 ($22.95 CAN)
1-55850-802-3, 288 pages

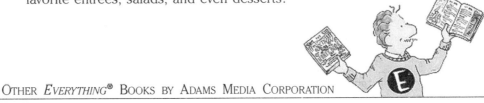

OTHER *EVERYTHING*® BOOKS BY ADAMS MEDIA CORPORATION

BUSINESS

Everything® **Business Planning Book**
Everything® **Coaching & Mentoring Book**
Everything® **Home-Based Business Book**
Everything® **Leadership Book**
Everything® **Managing People Book**
Everything® **Network Marketing Book**
Everything® **Online Business Book**
Everything® **Project Management Book**
Everything® **Selling Book**
Everything® **Start Your Own Business Book**
Everything® **Time Management Book**

COMPUTERS

Everything® **Build Your Own Home Page Book**
Everything® **Computer Book**

Everything® **Internet Book**
Everything® **Microsoft® Word 2000 Book**

COOKING

Everything® **Bartender's Book, $9.95**
Everything® **Barbecue Cookbook**
Everything® **Chocolate Cookbook**
Everything® **Cookbook**
Everything® **Dessert Cookbook**
Everything® **Diabetes Cookbook**
Everything® **Low-Carb Cookbook**
Everything® **Low-Fat High-Flavor Cookbook**
Everything® **Mediterranean Cookbook**
Everything® **One-Pot Cookbook**
Everything® **Pasta Book**
Everything® **Quick Meals Cookbook**
Everything® **Slow Cooker Cookbook**

Everything® **Soup Cookbook**
Everything® **Thai Cookbook**
Everything® **Vegetarian Cookbook**
Everything® **Wine Book**

HEALTH

Everything® **Anti-Aging Book**
Everything® **Dieting Book**
Everything® **Herbal Remedies Book**
Everything® **Hypnosis Book**
Everything® **Menopause Book**
Everything® **Stress Management Book**
Everything®**Vitamins, Minerals, and Nutritional Supplements Book**
Everything® **Nutrition Book**

HISTORY

Everything® **American History Book**

All Everything® books are priced at $12.95 or $14.95, unless otherwise stated. Prices subject to change without notice.
Canadian prices range from $11.95–$22.95 and are subject to change without notice.

Everything® **Civil War Book**
Everything® **World War II Book**

HOBBIES

Everything® **Bridge Book**
Everything® **Candlemaking Book**
Everything® **Casino Gambling Book**
Everything® **Chess Basics Book**
Everything® **Collectibles Book**
Everything® **Crossword and Puzzle Book**
Everything® **Digital Photography Book**
Everything® **Drums Book (with CD),**
  $19.95, ($31.95 CAN)
Everything® **Family Tree Book**
Everything® **Games Book**
Everything® **Guitar Book**
Everything® **Knitting Book**
Everything® **Magic Book**
Everything® **Motorcycle Book**
Everything® **Online Genealogy Book**
Everything® **Playing Piano and**
  Keyboards Book
Everything® **Rock & Blues Guitar**
  Book (with CD), $19.95,
  ($31.95 CAN)
Everything® **Scrapbooking Book**

HOME IMPROVEMENT

Everything® **Feng Shui Book**
Everything® **Gardening Book**
Everything® **Home Decorating Book**
Everything® **Landscaping Book**
Everything® **Lawn Care Book**
Everything® **Organize Your Home Book**

KIDS' STORY BOOKS

Everything® **Bedtime Story Book**
Everything® **Bible Stories Book**
Everything® **Fairy Tales Book**
Everything® **Mother Goose Book**

NEW AGE

Everything® **Astrology Book**

Everything® **Divining the Future Book**
Everything® **Dreams Book**
Everything® **Ghost Book**
Everything® **Meditation Book**
Everything® **Numerology Book**
Everything® **Palmistry Book**
Everything® **Spells and Charms Book**
Everything® **Tarot Book**
Everything® **Wicca and Witchcraft Book**

PARENTING

Everything® **Baby Names Book**
Everything® **Baby Shower Book**
Everything® **Baby's First Food Book**
Everything® **Baby's First Year Book**
Everything® **Breastfeeding Book**
Everything® **Get Ready for Baby Book**
Everything® **Homeschooling Book**
Everything® **Potty Training Book,**
  $9.95, ($15.95 CAN)
Everything® **Pregnancy Book**
Everything® **Pregnancy Organizer,**
  $15.00, ($22.95 CAN)
Everything® **Toddler Book**
Everything® **Tween Book**

PERSONAL FINANCE

Everything® **Budgeting Book**
Everything® **Get Out of Debt Book**
Everything® **Get Rich Book**
Everything® **Investing Book**
Everything® **Homebuying Book, 2nd Ed.**
Everything® **Homeselling Book**
Everything® **Money Book**
Everything® **Mutual Funds Book**
Everything® **Online Investing Book**
Everything® **Personal Finance Book**

PETS

Everything® **Cat Book**
Everything® **Dog Book**
Everything® **Dog Training and Tricks**
Everything® **Horse Book**
Everything® **Puppy Book**
Everything® **Tropical Fish Book**

REFERENCE

Everything® **Astronomy Book**
Everything® **Car Care Book**
Everything® **Christmas Book, $15.00,**
  ($21.95 CAN)
Everything® **Classical Mythology Book**
Everything® **Divorce Book**
Everything® **Etiquette Book**
Everything® **Great Thinkers Book**
Everything® **Learning French Book**
Everything® **Learning German Book**
Everything® **Learning Italian Book**
Everything® **Learning Latin Book**
Everything® **Learning Spanish Book**
Everything® **Mafia Book**
Everything® **Philosophy Book**
Everything® **Shakespeare Book**
Everything® **Tall Tales, Legends, &**
  Other Outrageous Lies Book
Everything® **Toasts Book**
Everything® **Trivia Book**
Everything® **Weather Book**
Everything® **Wills & Estate Planning**
  Book

RELIGION

Everything® **Angels Book**
Everything® **Buddhism Book**
Everything® **Catholicism Book**
Everything® **Judaism Book**
Everything® **Saints Book**
Everything® **World's Religions Book**
Everything® **Understanding Islam Book**

SCHOOL & CAREERS

Everything® **After College Book**
Everything® **College Survival Book**
Everything® **Cover Letter Book**
Everything® **Get-a-Job Book**
Everything® **Hot Careers Book**
Everything® **Job Interview Book**
Everything® **Online Job Search Book**
Everything® **Resume Book, 2nd Ed.**
Everything® **Study Book**

All Everything® books are priced at $12.95 or $14.95, unless otherwise stated. Prices subject to change without notice.
Canadian prices range from $11.95–$22.95 and are subject to change without notice.

WE HAVE EVERYTHING . . . .

SPORTS/FITNESS

Everything® **Bicycle Book**
Everything® **Fishing Book**
Everything® **Fly-Fishing Book**
Everything® **Golf Book**
Everything® **Golf Instruction Book**
Everything® **Pilates Book**
Everything® **Running Book**
Everything® **Sailing Book, 2nd Ed.**
Everything® **T'ai Chi and QiGong Book**
Everything® **Total Fitness Book**
Everything® **Weight Training Book**
Everything® **Yoga Book** ✎

TRAVEL

Everything® **Guide to Las Vegas**
Everything® **Guide to New England**
Everything® **Guide to New York City**
Everything® **Guide to Washington D.C.**

Everything® **Travel Guide to The Disneyland Resort®, California Adventure®, Universal Studios®, and the Anaheim Area**
Everything® **Travel Guide to the Walt Disney World® Resort, Universal Studios®, and Greater Orlando, 3rd Ed.**

WEDDINGS & ROMANCE

Everything® **Creative Wedding Ideas Book**
Everything® **Dating Book**
Everything® **Jewish Wedding Book**
Everything® **Romance Book**
Everything® **Wedding Book, 2nd Ed.**
Everything® **Wedding Organizer, $15.00 ($22.95 CAN)**

Everything® **Wedding Checklist, $7.95 ($11.95 CAN)**
Everything® **Wedding Etiquette Book, $7.95 ($11.95 CAN)**
Everything® **Wedding Shower Book, $7.95 ($12.95 CAN)**
Everything® **Wedding Vows Book, $7.95 ($11.95 CAN)**
Everything® **Weddings on a Budget Book, $9.95 ($15.95 CAN)**

WRITING

Everything® **Creative Writing Book**
Everything® **Get Published Book**
Everything® **Grammar and Style Book**
Everything® **Grant Writing Book**
Everything® **Guide to Writing Children's Books**
Everything® **Writing Well Book**

ALSO AVAILABLE:
THE EVERYTHING® KIDS' SERIES!

Each book is 8" x 9¼", 144 pages, and two-color throughout.

Everything® **Kids' Baseball Book, 2nd Edition, $6.95** ($11.95 CAN)
Everything® **Kids' Bugs Book, $6.95** ($10.95 CAN)
Everything® **Kids' Cookbook, $6.95** ($10.95 CAN)
Everything® **Kids' Joke Book, $6.95** ($10.95 CAN)
Everything® **Kids' Math Puzzles Book, $6.95** ($10.95 CAN)
Everything® **Kids' Mazes Book, $6.95** ($10.95 CAN)
Everything® **Kids' Money Book, $6.95** ($11.95 CAN)

Everything® **Kids' Monsters Book, $6.95** ($10.95 CAN)
Everything® **Kids' Nature Book, $6.95** ($11.95 CAN)
Everything® **Kids' Puzzle Book $6.95,** ($10.95 CAN)
Everything® **Kids' Science Experiments Book, $6.95** ($10.95 CAN)
Everything® **Kids' Soccer Book, $6.95** ($10.95 CAN)
Everything® **Kids' Travel Activity Book, $6.95** ($10.95 CAN)

Available wherever books are sold!
To order, call 800-872-5627, or visit us at everything.com

Everything® is a registered trademark of Adams Media Corporation.